THE EAGLE'S WAY

The Importance Of Love In Healthcare

Dr. Peter L. Johnston

Copyright 2023 by Dr. Peter L. Johnston

All rights reserved. This book or any portion thereof may not be reproduced or used in any manner whatsoever without the express written permission of the publisher except for the use of brief quotation in a book review.

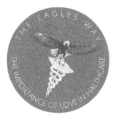

Eagle's Way Publishing

ISBN: 978-1-961416-37-6 (sc)
ISBN: 978-1-961416-38-3 (ebk)

CONTENTS

Preface 5

Introduction 7

Chapter 1: The Eagle's Way 13
Chapter 2: Fighting The Storm 26
Chapter 3: The Problems With Fighting 30
Chapter 4: Avoiding The Storm 49
Chapter 5: The Art Of Medicine 70
Chapter 6: An Age Of Separation 90
Chapter 7: The New Paradigm Of Consciousness 103
Chapter 8: The New Paradigm Of Mind And Matter 118
Chapter 9: The Re-Emergence Of Ancient Wisdom 135
Chapter 10: Embracing Illness 150
Chapter 11: Embracing The Non-Physical Causes Of Illness 172
Chapter 12: Embracing The Whole 185
Chapter 13: Nourishing The Body 197
Chapter 14: Love And Emotion In The New Paradigm 211
Chapter 15: Love And Healing In The New Paradigm 227
Chapter 16: The Scope Of Health Care 242
Chapter 17: Holistic Approach To Preventive Health 263
Chapter 18: Complementarity Of Orthodox
And Alternative Medicine 273
Chapter 19: Conclusion 282
Chapter 20: The Covid-19 Pandemic 293

Final Words 304
Endnotes 305
Glossary Of Therapies 330
Glossary Of Medical Terms 344

PREFACE

I n 1980, I referred three patients to a spiritual healer. One had metastatic cancer, another had rheumatoid arthritis and the third had an incurable lung disease. I had little to offer any of them. While spiritual healing seemed a long shot, there seemed little to lose by trying it. All three patients experienced "spontaneous remissions." One patient's arthritis subsided two days after he had hands-on healing. The patient with severe lung disease went close to death with a "healing reaction" before she achieved a remission that lasted thirteen years. The patient with metastatic cancer went into remission only after changing his job, sorting out his somewhat complicated love life, re-establishing a loving communication with his daughter and moving to a rural setting.

Being a conventional family practitioner, these results were mind-blowing. They led to a search for an understanding of how such miraculous events could occur. In the process of researching the subject, my previous understanding of 'mind' was indeed blown away and replaced by a far more expansive concept—that of the 'universal mind.' This book is about that journey.

As a general practitioner, I am by career and nature a generalist. I have no experience of academia and can claim no original research. My interest is in the big picture. If a specialist can be described as "one who knows more and more about less and less," I would describe myself as one who knows less and less about more and more. At least this is how it feels. The more I know, the more I realize I don't know.

I stand in awe at life itself and the incredible complexity of it all—yet its remarkable order.

I am very grateful to all the pioneers of the new frontier of consciousness—the scientists, psychologists, metaphysicians, philosophers, authors, and academics mentioned in this book. I am very grateful for the inspiration they have provided. I am very grateful to those I have directly quoted. The warmth and generosity with which they granted me permission to quote their words touched me deeply.

I want to give particular thanks to the wonderful people I have not thanked individually. Over forty years, patients, friends, authors, teachers, and workshop presenters have all contributed much to my education—and hence to this work.

Thanks to Dr. Andrew Horwood for his helpful advice. Thanks also to my family. My brother, Alan, sister Barb, son Mike, daughter Lara, and son-in-law, Toby Hemming helped with editing of the manuscript or gave advice. Special thanks go to my late brother-in-law, Bill Flynn, for his very valuable critique.

I am not sure who penned these words, but this line seems appropriate: "We teach best what we most need to learn."

Whoever it was, the words ring true. Writing this book has helped my understanding of life, love, and health. I trust it will help those who read it.

INTRODUCTION

In 1995, a senior colleague put this question to me. "Why are people choosing to use unproven remedies and unqualified healers when conventional scientific medicine can do more for people now than ever before?" His question was one of the triggers for writing this book.

This question is still being asked. Friends of Science in Medicine is a group of more than twelve hundred international scientists, clinicians and consumer advocates, whose main aim is to reverse the trend which sees government-funded institutions offering courses in healthcare sciences that are not underpinned by convincing scientific evidence. They believe that universities are places where good science should be promoted and defended. Professor Rob Morrison, a spokesman for the group, describes homeopathy, reflexology, energy medicine, tactile healing and kinesiology as "pseudoscience, quackery and nonsense".[1] The group has succeeded in closing half the 'pseudoscience' courses offered at British universities.[2]

The validity of the scientific method in establishing an evidence base for medicine is something I totally support. The profession should continue to make evidence-based medicine its standard and any healing therapy that fails to meet those standards should be excluded from accepted medical practice. However, that does not mean I support their exclusion from Universities. Far from it.

Research into medications is big business. Pharmaceutical companies conduct randomised double-blind trials to test any new drug.

Large numbers are given the new drug while similar numbers are given a placebo, an inert substance dressed up to look like the active drug. In a well conducted trial, neither the doctor nor patient knows which pill they are taking. If the results show that patients taking the new drug get significantly better results than the patients taking the placebo, the trial is deemed a success.

It may take a number of trials before a new drug can be considered both safe and therapeutically effective. Getting a new drug on to the market is an expensive exercise, frequently costing in excess of five hundred million dollars. The reward for success is a patent allowing the company a monopoly over the manufacture and distribution of the new drug for fifteen years. While this is an effective way of developing new medications, a patent does require the medication to be new. Patents cannot be applied to natural bodily components like vitamins, minerals and natural hormones.

A prime example is hormone replacement therapy. Pharmaceutical companies have marketed a number of synthetic hormones aimed at reducing the symptoms of menopause. They have been effective in reducing hot flushes but research two decades ago showed their usage to be associated with an increased rate of heart disease and strokes, sparking public interest in natural hormones.[3]

As a medical student I was complaining about having to grind powder with a mortar and pestle in a pharmacy prac class. At the time even pharmacists were rarely doing so as nearly all drugs were already manufactured and packaged ready for the shelf. Yet over the last twenty years, compounding pharmacies have sprung up to cater for this public demand. They produce not only the female sex hormones but also testosterone, thyroid hormones and melatonin, the latter being the hormone from the pineal gland. The mortar and pestle is back in action producing 'bio-identical' hormones in the form of creams, tablets, trochets and liquids.

Yet none of these bio-identical substances have been scientifically validated and government-funded bodies like universities need to research them, as private enterprise has no incentive to do so. I think it is important that all therapies be also given the opportunity to be used and researched in universities and teaching hospitals, because that is where the evidence base of any treatment can be tested.

Herbs have been used in Europe for centuries and there have been a large number of trials conducted.[4] Unfortunately, these trials lack the rigour of randomised double-blind trials but the prohibitive costs of such testing render it unlikely their efficacy will be proven to the standards required of medicine.

Probably the only way to prove that some of these therapies and substances work is to do 'outcome studies' whereby patients undergoing such therapies are compared with a control group.

Yet the very nature of natural healing complicates this process. Unlike antibiotics and medications, natural remedies rarely produce rapid cures or instant diminution of symptoms. More often clients undergo 'healing crises' which bring accentuation of their symptoms, after which they tend to improve. In other words, they get worse before they get better. Success is measured by the general direction of the illness rather than symptom relief. When healing is occurring, symptoms occur against a backdrop of increasing energy, wellbeing and optimism. When health is deteriorating, symptoms are more continuous and accompanied by a loss of energy and vitality.

Further complicating research is the tendency for natural therapists to combine treatments. It is not unusual for their clients to be having energy healing in the form of acupuncture or Bowen therapy and be taking herbs, homeopathic remedies and nutritional supplements, together with counselling. As often as not their clients will also be on medications from their doctor. Natural therapists also tend to change their regimes according to the client's progress. So it is nearly impossible to gauge the ingredient responsible for a successful outcome.

While acupuncture does have some scientific validation in terms of outcome studies,[5] its mechanism of action relies on a bio-energy the Chinese call 'chi'. At this time chi is not capable of being measured. Hence its existence and those of other bio-energies is questioned in scientific circles. Some bio-energetic therapies, like kinesiology, Emotional Freedom Technique (EFT), chakra readings and Reiki rely on gaining information from the client's subconscious, using methods considered too subjective to be accepted in the mainstream.

Many of the newer psychotherapies involve the psyche in its original definition of 'soul', referring to consciousness which survives death. Given that the soul can never be known objectively, it is hard to imagine these newer psychotherapies ever being welcomed into mainstream medicine.

In summary then, there is a large body of psychological, bio-energetic and physical healthcare therapies unproven—and possibly unprovable—to the level required by scientific medicine. These are all currently classified as CAM meaning 'alternative or complementary medicine'.

While I have made the generalization that Western Medicine is evidence based while CAM therapies lack this, it is not the complete truth. There are surgical procedures and medications, including anticancer drugs that have never been scientifically proven, while acupuncture, homeopathy, herbs and even prayer have had successful outcome studies, giving them some scientific credibility.[6,7,8,9]

This book aims to show that:

1. The difference between conventional and CAM therapies is as much philosophical as scientific.
2. Many alternative or complementary therapies, rather than representing a backward step, are products of a new scientific paradigm—and hence an evolutionary step forward.
3. It is a healthy development to have these two systems of healthcare operating separately and
4. Both systems are essential and complement each other.

In the process of exploring the underlying philosophy of CAM, the shortcomings of conventional medicine will be outlined but this should not be taken as a criticism of scientific medicine, which I have spent most of my life practicing. Even though I have been utilizing CAM approaches for forty years, most my consultations have involved orthodox medicine. The benefits of conventional medicine are so obvious as to preclude the need for justification. This is not

THE EAGLE'S WAY

the case with CAM therapies. While a large section of the general public has accepted them, the scientific and medical community question their benefits. Having personally experienced the benefits of CAM, I have a special interest in trying to understand the ways in which they work. Over the past forty years it has been of great benefit for me to be able to refer patients to CAM practitioners when they were suffering from conditions for which conventional medicine has no cure.

CHAPTER 1

The Eagle's Way

In 1920, when my father worked as an intern at the Perth Public Hospital, the acute wards were largely occupied by patients with typhoid and diphtheria. Mostly children and young adults, many did not survive, as there were no really effective antibacterial medications. In fact, there are few therapies from that era still in use today.

A Truly Creative Era for Medicine

The period between 1940 and 1980 was a remarkably fertile one for medicine. Compared to my father, who must have felt relatively powerless to help his young patients, I am extremely grateful to have entered the medical profession in the midst of its most creative era.

Infection and Inflammation

In 1941, the year I was born, penicillin was used for the first time on a patient. While the patient ultimately died, his initial response was so dramatic that it ushered in the antibiotic era, which transformed the treatment of infection. Previously fatal diseases like pneumonia, septicaemia, and meningitis could now be cured. Also, by treating scarlet fever and primary syphilis, previously fatal chronic disease in the form of rheumatic heart disease and tertiary syphilis could be averted.

DR. PETER L. JOHNSTON

Within twenty-five years, more than twenty antibiotics were discovered and developed. Among these were streptomycin, isoniazid and rifampicin. While improved sanitation and the practice of isolating patients with tuberculosis in sanatoria had reduced the incidence of TB during the first half of the twentieth century, the arrival of these antibiotics made such inroads on this old enemy that by 1980, tuberculosis had almost disappeared from the Western world. Unfortunately, the arrival of AIDS has allowed some resurfacing of this chronic illness.

Prevention of infection in the Western world started with Jenner's cowpox vaccine against smallpox in 1796. Almost a century later, Louis Pasteur produced a vaccine against rabies. Typhoid, diphtheria, and tetanus vaccines followed in the early twentieth century. The Second World War brought a more active focus on immunization, and during this golden medical era, vaccines against polio, measles, mumps, rubella, hepatitis A and B, meningitis, and pneumonia were produced. With the founding of the World Health Organization in the post-war period, global vaccination programs began. The most notable success was the total eradication of smallpox—the last case was recorded in 1977.

Where no microbe can be found or identified, inflammation can be suppressed by cortisone, which was discovered and synthesized in 1949. A natural hormone secreted by the adrenal gland, it has proven to be life-saving in asthma, Addison's disease, systemic lupus, ulcerative colitis, croup, and anaphylactic shock. In the form of creams and eye drops, it provides dramatic improvement in many diseases of the skin and eyes.

Resuscitation

At the height of the polio epidemic in 1952, the Blegdam Hospital in Copenhagen was overwhelmed with up to fifty children arriving daily and with only seven respirators available. An anaesthetist suggested doing tracheotomies on all of them, attaching tubing and bags, and asking medical students to squeeze the bags and breathe for them until their respiratory muscles recovered. By the time the epidemic

THE EAGLE'S WAY

was over, 1,500 medical students (on six-hour shifts) had worked 165,000 hours and reduced the mortality rate of polio from over 90 per cent to 25 per cent.[1] Within a few years, 'assisted ventilation' had become a central feature in caring for the seriously ill.

In the late 1940s, paediatricians found they could resuscitate babies by using mouth-to-mouth breathing. Later, it was used on adults, especially in drowning accidents. Defibrillation was first used directly on the heart in 1947 and was later found to be effective just by being applied to the outer chest wall. In 1966, the combination of rhythmic pressure to the chest wall with mouth-to-mouth breathing was endorsed at an international conference. By 1968, we were busy learning these skills, which came to be called CPR (cardiopulmonary resuscitation), and using defibrillation along with it. When I worked at Royal Perth Hospital in 1968, nobody died—they had cardiac arrests until we gained some efficiency with the procedure.

Nowadays, not only is CPR used by doctors and ambulance personnel, but it is also taught to the general public. In an emergency, CPR has been amply demonstrated to save lives by maintaining circulation and oxygenation until defibrillation is available. Defibrillators are frequently available at sporting and other public venues. CPR is especially important for young people with no history of heart disease, whose hearts have stopped because of drowning or electrocution.

Replacing Organ Function

Fortunately, polio is uncommon these days. Lung function is more often compromised by head or chest injuries or by major surgery to the chest and abdomen. Keeping these patients in intensive care on a respirator until they can breathe on their own is life-saving.

In 1944, the artificial kidney was invented. Now called dialysis, it has saved the lives of many people suffering from acute kidney failure, allowing time for them to recover from their illness. For those with more serious, progressive kidney disease, dialysis keeps them alive while they await kidney transplantation.

DR. PETER L. JOHNSTON

The creation of the heart-lung machine in 1955 initiated the era of open-heart surgery. Now referred to as 'bypass', the machine takes over the function of the heart and lungs, allowing the surgeon to repair valves, congenital malformations, and coronary artery disease.

Surgery

In the early 1930s, my mother used to enjoy assisting a prominent general surgeon who would tie off blood vessels with his thumb and first two fingers and use his ring and little fingers to cut the ties with scissors. Such a skill was very valuable in an era when reducing blood loss was crucial. Blood transfusion became a much safer procedure after the Rhesus factor was discovered in 1942.

Curare was used for centuries by South American tribes to tip arrows, but its capacity for paralysing its victims was utilized in the 1940s to provide deep relaxation for abdominal surgery. It also allowed lower concentrations of anaesthetic to be used, which led to a new range of anaesthetics.

Using the operating microscope, which came into use in 1954, surgeons can cure otosclerosis, a form of hereditary deafness. They can also cure blindness due to cataracts, and small blood vessels can also be repaired, allowing severed limbs to be reattached and lethal brain aneurysms to be removed.

Harold Hopkins, a brilliant optical physicist, invented the fully flexible fibre-optic endoscope in 1954. Capable of shedding light in all directions, it enabled doctors to view the stomach, duodenum, and large bowel in their entirety. It also allowed exploration of the bladder and lungs.

A few years later, he invented the laparoscope. One of the earliest surgeons to utilize the new technology was Patrick Steptoe, a gynaecologist who used it to harvest mature eggs. In collaboration with Bob Edwards, he produced the first test-tube baby. Not long after, surgeons were removing gall bladders and exploring the abdomen via the laparoscope, while orthopaedic surgeons were exploring knees and shoulders.

THE EAGLE'S WAY

Charnley did his first hip replacement in 1961, but the procedure was not used widely until the 1970s.

Imaging and Interventional Radiology

X-rays came into use in the early twentieth century and were used to create images of the bony skeleton. In the 1950s, contrast agents were discovered, which allowed X-rays to show images of the bowel, kidneys, bladder, and salivary glands.

Ultrasound was first used in 1942 but required much refining and experimentation before it came into general use in the 1970s. In the same decade, CT (computed tomography) scanning produced images of cross sections of the body before MRI (magnetic resonance imaging) brought lifelike images of bodily organs without using X-radiation.

Although angiography was first used in 1927, it was the invention of the Seldinger technique in 1953 that made it a relatively risk-free procedure. Not only could blood vessels be imaged, but probes could also be passed along the vessels, obstructions removed, and the vessels kept patent (open) by the insertion of mechanical devices called stents.

Medications

The era between 1940 and 1980 produced the bulk of all the medications now used in medicine. Antibiotics, cortisone, and new anaesthetics have already been mentioned. Medications to help high blood pressure, rheumatoid arthritis and degenerative joint disease, Parkinson's disease, migraine, epilepsy, gout, haemophilia, and childhood leukaemia were discovered. Psychiatric medications to treat depression, anxiety, bipolar disorder, and psychoses also came into use in the 1950s and 1960s, and of course, the contraceptive pill gave women some realistic control over family planning and made a significant contribution to the sexual revolution.

DR. PETER L. JOHNSTON

The Decline of Scientific Optimism

This golden era had seen great advances in medicine, surgery, and obstetrics. In the field of life-saving surgery and resuscitation, progress was dramatic. In the 1960s, there was a feeling of optimism that science and technology would find a cure for all ailments confronting humanity. The first heart transplant had taken place in 1968. Successful kidney transplants had occurred. New antibiotics were still being found, and new medications for mental disease were being hailed as breakthroughs in the treatment of depression and anxiety. It was an exciting time in medicine.

Significant scientific developments have continued to occur, and surgical techniques have certainly continued to evolve. Yet it seems to me that those great expectations waned from the high point of the sixties. Maybe the increasing awareness of drug side-effects contributed? Perhaps the failure to make significant progress toward a cure for cancer despite vast expenditure on research showed a limitation to the scientific medical frontier?

The medical breakthroughs of the golden era spawned a new range of specialists to use the developed drugs and technologies but produced fewer doctors interested in scientific research. Between 1968 and 1978, the number of doctors undertaking postdoctoral research in the United States decreased by half.[2] The number of new medications was averaging about seventy per year in the 1960s, but by 1971, this was down to less than thirty a year and has stayed around that level ever since.[3] Furthermore, many of the drugs introduced after 1970 were more expensive variations of treatments for diseases already addressed by older medications.

At the same time, alternative health-care systems were emerging and growing in popularity in the Western world. From the 1960s, there has been a steady flow of new, alternative therapies along with a revival of interest in ancient systems of healing.

The Growth of Alternative Therapies

The words *alternative* and *complementary* are used to describe unconventional or nonmainstream medical therapies. The *Oxford Dictionary* defines *complementary medicine* as "medical therapy that falls beyond the scope of scientific medicine, but which may be used alongside it in the treatment of disease and ill health."

As there is no viable alternative to conventional medicine for acute or emergency conditions, the word 'complementary' better describes the function of alternative medicine as an adjunct to mainstream approaches. Over recent years, *CAM* has come into use as an acronym referring to 'complementary and alternative medicine'. In the course of this book, all three words may be used to describe therapies considered to be outside mainstream scientific medicine.

Statistics suggest people are indeed turning to alternative remedies and healers. In Australia, people are spending more money on various forms of "alternative medicine" than they are spending on pharmaceuticals.[4,5] The trend is similar in the United States and Europe.[6,7,8,9,10]

Possible Reasons for the Rise of CAM Therapies

1. The relative safety of natural therapeutic agents

One of the reasons for the increasing popularity of alternative approaches and supplements is a growing awareness of the side effects of conventional medicines. The powerful nature of pharmaceutical drugs and their potential for side effects requires physicians to warn patients about undesirable outcomes. Unfortunately, by the power of suggestion, such negative information tends to increase the incidence of unwanted outcomes.

On the other hand, there is a perception that alternative medicines are more natural and safe. In truth, herbs, like any naturally growing plant, may be quite toxic.[11] However, taken as a broad generalisation, there is truth in this perception. CAM medicines are more natural.

Vitamins and minerals exist naturally in the human body. Herbs grow in nature and are milder in their actions than drugs derived from the same source. So while the therapeutic potency of herbs might be less than that of pharmaceutical drugs, their side effects are also less potent.

2. The growth of the green movement

As a school student in the 1950s, our teachers inspired us with the idea of science being not only exciting but also heroic. The forces of nature were something to be tamed and conquered. Since then, awareness of the environment has grown. We have become aware of the extent to which we have polluted and poisoned the land, air, and waters of our planet with our uncontrolled approach to science and technology. The attitude of 'progress at all costs' has been all too prevalent in the Western world. Addressing the needs of our planet is now understood to be the responsible course of action. This shift in attitude may have influenced our approach to personal health as well as planetary health. Faith in the ability of science and technology to solve the problems of life appears to have diminished. The move toward 'green' movements and away from chemical and inorganic solutions may be a second reason for the popularity of CAM therapies.[12,13]

3. The length of consultations

With advances in medical technology, medical practitioners are capable of making more exact diagnoses by using imaging and pathology tests. There is less need to take a long history and do a thorough physical examination. As a result, consultations have become shorter and may compare unfavourably with the long consultations of most alternative practitioners.

4. The prevalence of chronic disease

The advances in medical science have brought about a significant increase in life expectancy. The average woman in Australia can expect to live into her mid-eighties and the average man make it into his early eighties. This longer lifespan brings with it more chronic disorders. CAM therapies can offer hope in this area. Their accent on lifestyle changes often appeal to patients with chronic illnesses, especially if they're unable to get relief with their medical treatments. Acupuncture has shown some success in helping relieve chronic pain.[14] The use of long-term opioids in coping with chronic pain is an escalating problem. Morphine and codeine have been traditionally used but have been shown to give only partial relief from ongoing pain. All too soon patients become addicted to these drugs. And over the past few years the number of deaths from accidental overdoses from these medications is skyrocketing. So as a profession, we doctors are desperately searching for adequate substitutes, and acupuncture is one of the more promising.

5. A renewed respect for tradition

As a young GP, I enthusiastically prescribed every new drug as soon as it came onto the market. However, I have become more conservative with age. All too often, the exciting new drug proved to have unacceptable side effects but it took some years for these to emerge. As a result, I have tended to stay with the medications that have stood the test of time.

Perhaps this principle has guided others. If a healing system or an herb has been used for centuries, presumably it has worked for some. While not scientifically verified, its long-standing use may constitute a reason for people to give it a try.

6. Treating the patient rather than the disease

Complementary therapists claim to be treating the patient rather than the disease. Instead of fighting disease, they are supporting the patient and helping to fortify him or her. Nutritionists and naturopaths tend to give their support at physical levels. Homeopaths, kinesiologists, and Reiki practitioners are giving their support with subtle energies. Psychotherapists are giving support at mental and emotional levels, while some practitioners may be lending support at all levels. Overall, the focus is one of interest in the client's life, which can be comforting.

7. Holistic or Integrative Medicine

There are also medical and alternative practitioners who attract clients who are seeking meaning in their lives. While their clients might present problems that are physical, mental, or emotional, holistic practitioners encourage exploration into what might be underlying their clients' symptoms. Why has this affliction hit now? Is it trying to communicate something? What can one do to lead a healthy, joyful, and purposeful life? How can one use this health crisis to make changes to empower one's life? These are questions about life and its meaning. While they could be described as philosophical, they are often more spiritual. When illness threatens the quality or quantity of one's life, the question of meaning is not just one of academic curiosity. Even when the search for meaning is devoid of any religious input, it is still a spiritual pursuit.

Those therapists whose focus is on treating the whole person—body, mind, emotions, and spirit—call themselves *holistic practitioners*. Some medical practitioners combine conventional medicine, alternative therapies, and a holistic approach. When doing so, they categorize themselves as practitioners of *holistic medicine* or *integrative medicine*.

8. A Deeper Transition

The more I thought about this issue, the more it seemed to reflect a deeper shift. Whereas the underlying *modus operandi* of conventional medicine is to fight disease, alternative and holistic treatments lack this aggressive approach.

In general, alternative therapies do not fight disease. The common philosophy shared by CAM therapies as a whole is one of support and nurturing. Whether by offering more time, natural remedies, relaxing massage, sweet-smelling aromas, or deep and meaningful counselling, CAM therapists are attempting to support the aggregate of body, mind, emotions, and soul. Fighting or avoiding the problem is not the aim, because the problem is not usually the focus of attention. The focus is on strengthening the client's organs or defence system. Or it may be helping to provide insight, motivation, and faith to aid the healing process.

The Eagle and Its Way

In ancient times, the symbol for trouble was the *storm*. We still speak about stormy weather and stormy times (e.g., stormy marriages, stormy moods, and stormy relationships). The word conjures up black clouds, dark skies, lightning, thunder, and driving rain. While rain may symbolise tears and sadness, thunder and lightning have an angrier, more threatening, and dangerous symbolism. The dark clouds, with their foreboding nature, are often used to describe depression. The *storm* has served well as a symbol for the problems of life and the emotions that go with them. In the health arena, these are the diseases and disordered emotional states that afflict the lives of so many.

On the other hand, the symbol for freedom from trouble was the *bird*. Birds are the only creatures capable of leaving the earth. We still use the expression "free as a bird" as a metaphor for leaving our troubles behind.

However, if birds actually fly into storms, most do not find total freedom, as they cannot make much headway. More often they deal with storms by using other means.

Fighting the storm is one approach. Birds will point their beaks into a storm, flap their wings harder, and do their best to counter the difficult conditions. As a result, they do make some headway toward their intended destination but tend to get a bit knocked about in the process.

If the battering gets too much for them, an alternative is *avoiding* the storm. By seeking more sheltered areas, they manage to survive but make little progress toward their destination.

The bird that demonstrates the most practical option is the eagle. It flies *into* and *through* the dark clouds, elevates itself above the storm, and flies unhindered to its destination.

Fighting and avoidance are natural responses to fear. 'Fight or flight' is part of our animal instinct for survival. While the eagle confronts the storm, its approach is not to fight it or avoid it. The eagle accepts the presence of the black clouds, goes through them, and heads for its destination.

Application of Eagle's Way to Health Care

I see the eagle as a metaphor for an emerging approach to healing— one based on accepting illness rather than fighting or avoiding it. There is an underlying philosophy in holistic medicine that goes something like this:

> Despite appearances to the contrary, life has an underlying order to it. Science is about understanding the laws guiding this natural order. There is a similar underlying purpose in every individual life. While the purpose may change as people grow, living in accordance with one's purpose brings inner peace. Just as a bird is happy flying, so people are happy when they are exercising their talents and abilities in productive ways. When people are happy and following their hearts' desires, health tends to follow.

Mainstream Western medicine, with its advanced scientific and technological complexity, operates predominantly at the level of fighting disease. Holistic medicine, instead of fighting illness, embraces it. Just as a storm may bring life-giving rain, disease may bring a life-giving message.

The word *disease* originated from the Old French *desaise,* meaning a 'lack of ease.'[15] Disease, when explored in depth, may be found to involve repressed emotions, unacknowledged fears, unconscious beliefs, or disowned aspects of one's personality. In other words, the underlying cause of disease can be a disconnection

THE EAGLE'S WAY

from aspects of oneself, a loss of something needed for completeness, or a lack of wholeness.

The holistic approach to health care is not about removing anything. It is all about restoring something. It is not about fighting any aspect of the self. It is focused on embracing and accepting one's self fully, regardless of what one might regard as one's flaws or deficiencies. By finding and restoring what is missing, one can move toward wholeness. The words *whole, holy, heal,* and *health* all came from the same Germanic root derivation.[16] Every healing event creates more wholeness and raises the level of self-awareness, thereby increasing the degree of inner freedom and capacity for joy in life. It could almost be a description of flying.

CHAPTER 2

Fighting The Storm

n contrast with some Eastern systems of medicine[1] that focus on health and what contributes to being healthy, Western medicine has focused on disease. Once dissection of the dead became permissible, physicians examined cadavers and rapidly established an accurate map of human anatomy. From this base, they gradually gathered an impressive knowledge of disease. Out of this understanding came a system for fighting pain, death, disease, and suffering unequalled in human history.

Surgery

Not surprisingly, surgery has been the fastest growing area of health care. The simplest way of dealing with disease is to remove the diseased part. Diseased tissue on the skin and accessible areas can be removed with little inconvenience. Tonsils, adenoids, and appendixes can also be excised with no obvious ill effects. Removal of the gall bladder leaves the body without a reservoir for bile, but this deficiency can be managed by changing to a low-fat diet. Because the body can cope adequately with only one kidney, ovary, testicle, and lung, removal of one of these paired organs is safe, provided that the remaining organ is functioning normally.

THE EAGLE'S WAY

In hollow organs like the bowel and bladder, removal of the diseased section and rearrangement of the remaining tissue are commonplace, allowing organs to be reconstructed in a functional way. One of my patients, who had a large bladder cancer, successfully used a reconstructed bladder for more than ten years. In similar fashion, plastic surgeons can remove skin blemishes and wrinkles, rearranging the skin in creative ways to fight the ravages of time.

However, the greatest advance in surgery has been the replacement of diseased parts with either mechanical devices or grafts. Prosthetic hip joints, knee joints, and heart valves are now commonly implanted. The bionic ear, a complex and brilliant invention, is coming into more use. *Homografts*, ranging from skin grafts to coronary bypass, are taken from a different area of the same patient. *Heterografts*, such as kidneys, corneas, liver, and bone marrow, come from donors who are either living or recently deceased.

In short, surgery fights disease by removing the diseased tissue and reconstructing the body in the most effective way to repair the damage and cover the loss. Creative and life-saving as it is, surgery treats disease as an enemy against which it wages war. The surgeon's role is to eliminate the enemy, patch up the wounded, and clear the battlefield of casualties.

Medicine

Medicine is defined as the science and practice of diagnosis, treatment, and prevention of disease. Within the medical profession, this definition excludes surgery. In medicine, the major battle is fought with medication.

A brief look at some of the categories of medication allows a glimpse of the fighting qualities intended. *Anti*biotics, *anti*fungals, *anti*helmintics, and *anti*viral agents attack parasitic external invaders. *Anti*-cancer drugs attack the internal invader. *Anti*emetics and *anti*diarrhoeal agents combat symptoms, while *anti*convulsants and *anti*-migraine preparations mitigate and help prevent attacks of epilepsy and migraine. *Anti*histamines reduce the impact of allergies, and *anti*-Parkinsonian drugs and *anti*diabetic agents help combat the manifestations of disease.[2]

In general, the policy with medications is to use the lowest dose of a drug capable of generating the desired result. The more lethal the disease, the more the physician needs to use powerful drugs. Radiation, a heavy weapon in the fight against cancer, tends to be used in the same way. The more serious the situation, the higher the dosage required.

In preventive medicine, the most successful technique has been immunisation, sometimes called vaccination. A tiny dose of dead pathogenic microorganisms—or an even tinier dose of living germs of similar nature to the pathogens—is administered to the patient. Feeling under attack, the patient's defence system starts manufacturing antibodies against these microorganisms. Antibodies are like guided missiles, specifically targeting potential invaders. Having an arsenal of antibodies prevents particular invaders gaining a foothold in the body.

So, while medication is primarily aimed at fighting disease, disorders, and symptoms, immunisation is aimed at boosting the fighting power of the body. Combat is the essence of each form of treatment.

Psychiatry

As in the treatment of physical ailments, the mainstay of treatment in mainstream psychiatry is drug therapy. Psychotropic medications are aimed at attacking the problems with a range of weapons. Antidepressants are used against depression. Anxiolytic agents are used against anxiety states, and antipsychotic medications are used to combat psychoses.[3]

Electroconvulsive therapy, otherwise known as ECT or shock therapy, is used to fight severe depression by giving the patient a brief epileptic fit. It first came into use in 1938 when it was thought epilepsy sufferers did not get symptoms of schizophrenia and depression. As antidepressant medications became more popular, ECT has been confined to use in severe depression and situations where medication has failed.

Behavioural therapy is another mainstream treatment that aims to eradicate undesirable habits, such as smoking, substance abuse, or overeating, without using drugs. The strategy can involve a battle against the old behaviour. While I was working as an intern, I visited a small movie theatre used for aversion therapy. Each seat was wired for the patient to receive a small electric charge each time an inappropriate slide was shown. For the smoker, the slide might be a cigarette advertisement. For the alcoholic, an image of a beer might elicit a mini shock.

Emergency Medicine

This is an area where vast improvements have occurred. In 1969, when I was working in a military hospital in South Vietnam, a seriously wounded soldier could be lifted by helicopter, receive intravenous fluids while in the aircraft, be brought to the military hospital, be resuscitated, and be in the operating theatre within half an hour of his injury. As a result, soldiers survived injuries that would have been fatal in any other era. One person who has been coming to see me as a patient for thirty years lost both legs and his right arm; however, he has remained fully employed, raised a family, and became an inspiration to many.

The 1960s saw some of the greatest advances in resuscitation—in fact, it could be described as a time of great enthusiasm and optimism in our quest to overcome death and prolong life.

Here in Australia in 1972, I heard Bill Hayden, federal minister for health, state that 70 per cent of our total health expenditure was spent on people who "wouldn't be here in twelve months." It is estimated that 10 to 15 per cent of the US health budget is spent on the last month of life.[4] Although this figure may be slowly moderating, there still seems to be an attitude of fighting to the death—a preference for heroic, last-ditch stands.

CHAPTER 3

The Problems With Fighting

While fighting diseases brings considerable benefits to patients in curing diseases and alleviating symptoms, it does have some drawbacks. The shortcomings of fighting come under three headings: metaphysical, philosophical, and practical.

A. The Metaphysical Problem with Fighting

Metaphysics derives from the Greek word meaning "beyond physics." Since the time of the classical Greek philosophers Plato and Aristotle, metaphysicians have grappled with the relationship between thoughts and physical substance, between the world of ideas and the world of the senses. Our senses are limited in terms of what they can take in. Visible light makes up only a small fragment of the known range of the electromagnetic spectrum. The vast range of waves, including X-rays, microwaves, radio waves, television waves, and cosmic waves, lies in the invisible ultraviolet or infrared range. Sound waves that are audible to the human ear are also limited. Dogs and dolphins can hear sounds that humans cannot.

Sensory limitation resulted in difficulty accepting the concept of the earth being round. The earth still seems flat to my senses, but then I have learned that my senses deceive me. The pen in my hand appears to be shiny, blue, smooth, and solid. Yet under a microscope,

THE EAGLE'S WAY

the surface is no longer smooth and shiny but rough and dull. As to its solidity, scientists tell us it is more than 99 per cent empty space. Finally, its blue colour disappears when the lights go out. The colour is in the light, not the pen.

As I understand metaphysics, thought is the creator of matter and experience. Before a house is built, it is first a design, a drawing of a plan. Prior to the plan, it is a vision in the architect's mind. The actions we take in our lives primarily derive from our intentions and thoughts. Thoughts emanate from our conscious mind if we have consciously planned them. Or they come from our subconscious mind, if it is a habitual, instinctive, or absent-minded one.

The brain and consciousness

To get to the ultimate cause of disease, we need to go beyond the senses. Some philosophers and scientists see matter as the fundamental basis of reality. To them, consciousness and thought arise in an evolutionary process as a result of brain development in mankind. Certainly, the brains of Neanderthal and Cro-Magnon humans differ from those of our current *Homo sapiens*. Anthropological research has not yet clarified the time span over which human consciousness might have evolved.

Others, myself included, see it entirely from the opposite direction. For us, consciousness is the fundamental basis of life. The mind is the creator; matter is the creation. Before the material world came into being, there was creative thought. For the metaphysician, the body did not develop a consciousness through a process of evolution. Pre-existing consciousness clothed itself in a body and adapted the body to its environment in an evolutionary fashion. Anthropology and metaphysics both see the body evolving, but each discipline sees a different causal factor underlying that evolution.

Unlike the brain, consciousness is not limited to the confines of the skull. Thoughts can travel to the ends of the earth and beyond. If I want to reflect on my holiday in Fiji, my mind can be there in an instant. It can travel back in time and space, but my body and brain do not travel there.

I believe that consciousness is unlimited in time and space. The brain on the other hand is finite matter. I see the brain as being like a transmission station for the mind—the individual instrument of the mind in this three-dimensional world. It receives energy waves, sometimes called vibrations, from this three-dimensional realm and passes them on to the mind, which can digest them and then make decisions. The mind then passes the information back to the brain, which organizes the execution of the task. In addition, the brain oversees the subconscious functions of metabolism, growth, and body function. The brain is a marvellous instrument, but it is not the creator of human life. Life exists in the fertilized cell and the foetus before the brain comes into being. Yet the remarkable transformation from one cell into a human form is guided by a formless intelligence, which I refer to as consciousness or mind.

The self-fulfilling nature of belief

Beliefs have a tendency to be self-fulfilling. It might be easier to understand this by using an example. Take a young boy who is afraid of dogs. The boy has a belief that dogs are dangerous. He is afraid a dog might bite him. When he meets a dog, this belief comes very much to the forefront. Fear arises. This fear has an impact, both inside and outside the child. Internally, it might produce discomfort in the child's solar plexus, the so-called 'butterflies in the stomach.' He might also feel dryness in the mouth and an acute sense of discomfort. These are indications that his adrenal glands are on full alert and are providing the energy for the fight or flight needed in this situation.

The dog picks up the fear as an energy or vibration and feels a similar desire to fight or take flight. Its own welfare is endangered. If it decides attack is the best means of defence, it will snarl at the lad and possibly bite him. The end result will be a strengthening of the initial belief about all dogs being dangerous. This creates a vicious circle in which the belief gets stronger with each negative experience.

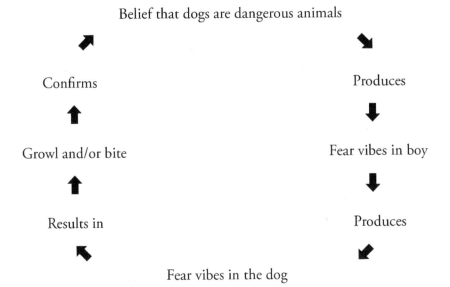

This vicious cycle cannot be resolved at the physical level. It is not realistic to completely exclude dogs from the child's environment. The problem will continue because the problem does not lie with the dog. It lies with the child's belief system. Another child who believes dogs to be loyal, fun-loving creatures might have the same dog wagging its tail and eating out of her hand. An outsider might see the same dog interacting differently with two children; but to the two participants, they would be seeing two entirely different animals.

How we actually see

Our eyes are like cameras. They faithfully record everything we see—exactly as it is. Nevertheless, that is not what we actually see. What the eye records is light. If there is no light present, all we see is a blackish hue regardless of what colour the object might be. When light is present, it reflects off all objects, creating the colours and shapes of the images that flow into our eyes. As the light traverses the lens of the eye, the image is inverted and absorbed by the retina, the light-sensitive layer at the back of the eye. From there, the image travels around both sides of the brain through a number of synapses to the area of the brain called the optic cortex.

The optic cortex is where visual memory is thought to be stored. In this journey, the image is somehow processed through a "bio-computer," which poses these types of questions:

- Is this scene or image familiar?
- Where have I seen this before?
- Have I got a name or label for this?
- Does it interest me?
- Do I really want to see it?
- What do I expect to see here?
- What do I believe about this scene?

These thoughts, desires, beliefs, interests, or aversions impact the original image and colour the whole picture. In a matter of milliseconds, the end product is returned to the eyes and projected forth. *And that is what we actually see.*

This is the reason two critics can see the same play and describe it so differently that you wonder whether they are talking about the same production. When I visit patients in their homes I tend to notice their books—or the absence of them. I take in little of the decor or furniture. Other doctors may notice the colour scheme, furnishings, or the dust level. People tend to notice what interests them. Toddlers, being so open, notice insects and objects that I don't see. What we see is not the totally external phenomenon we assume it to be. In reality, the experience is as much an internal one. What we see "out there" actually reflects what we are inside. In the Talmud, one of the sacred books of the Jewish people, this quotation is found: "*We do not see things as they are. We see things as we are.*"

If that lad acquires a dog of his own and learns to love it, his fear will tend to diminish and the appreciation he has for his dog will transfer to dogs in a more general sense. So when he meets other dogs, they will tend to behave differently. He will no longer need to fight them or avoid them. Like an eagle, he will have addressed the problem and risen above that particular storm.

THE EAGLE'S WAY

The metaphysics of health

In understanding the way thoughts and beliefs create experiences, it is easier to understand what thoughts and beliefs can do to the physical body. When people are angry, some show it by acting out with arms flailing, voice raised, face red and flushed. Others may try to suppress the anger. But the pursed lip, set jaw, and lack of speech or spontaneity may still convey the impression of anger as strong emotions are difficult to conceal.

How do emotions affect the body over a lifetime? The most accessible is facial expression. We use the terms "frown lines" and "smile lines" to describe the visible signs informing the observer of the dominant way in which a person has viewed his or her life. The lines give an indication as to whether a person has experienced life as a hard road or a fun run.

If emotions and beliefs affect facial skin, perhaps it is not such a big jump to suggest that other organs might be similarly affected. This is my understanding of metaphysics as applied to health. If a thought brings a sense of happiness, unity, belonging, and security, it results in a positive emotion like love or joy. If a thought brings a sense of conflict, unhappiness, insecurity, or separation, then the result will be a negative emotion like fear, anger, or sadness.

If negative emotions are experienced at the time, the energy attached to them is released. However, if the emotions are too overwhelming or traumatic to be experienced fully they remain within. Like a beach ball being held underwater, it takes energy to keep emotions from floating to the surface. When people's energy levels are low, these painful emotions and sometimes memories will tend to arise. However, if these emotions are repressed for years, they seem to either deplete energy, or the energy seems to turn inward and affect the host physically.

What actually happens in terms of the pathogenic process is not yet clear. The relatively new science of psycho-neuro-immunology is researching this connection between emotions and disease.

Fighting disease does not always address the deeper causes.

The metaphysician sees disease as a projection of the individual's inner world. Like a movie, the picture is occurring out there on the screen, but its source is the film inside the projector. Fighting disease is fighting the outcome rather than the cause. It corresponds to fixing the movie screen when the problem lies with the film. Nevertheless, the senses see only the physical outcome. Orthodox medicine is based on science, which values careful observation. In general, this leads to disease being viewed as a physical phenomenon and treated accordingly.

A cosmetic surgeon can remove the furrows from a patient's forehead with a facelift. Nevertheless, those furrows will return as long as the patient continues to worry and age. Like the bird fighting the storm, the surgery produces a temporary benefit, but the patient can also experience some undesirable effects from the surgical procedure.

From the metaphysical perspective, accepting a disease as incurable or fatal is giving it unwarranted power. While it may indeed turn out to be incurable or lethal, it is worth exploring one's inner world before accepting such an outcome as inevitable. Chronic disease may be the result of an inner conflict that can be addressed. Seeking the deeper causes of disease is akin to entering the storm clouds. Rather than fighting or avoiding disease, the patient embraces the problem and explores its meaning with a view to rising above the storm, resolving the inner conflict and finding a higher purpose.

B. The Philosophical Problem with Fighting

To every action, there is an equal and opposite reaction.
—Isaac Newton

All suffering is caused by our cravings.
—second noble truth of Buddha

What you resist persists.
—major principle of yoga

Resist not evil.
—Matthew 5:39

THE EAGLE'S WAY

The major philosophical disciplines advise against fighting problems. In the sixth century BC, Gautama Siddhartha, known as the Buddha, proclaimed his four noble truths. In saying that all suffering was caused by our cravings, he expanded it by explaining that craving was of two main kinds: craving to have what we do not have and craving not to have what we do have. This latter statement is what we do when we fight disease. We crave not to have it. We fight to get rid of it. The Buddha's advice was to detach from this craving and follow the eightfold noble path.

About six centuries later, the evangelist Matthew quoted Jesus of Nazareth, recommending that we not resist evil. Two thousand years ago, the people of Palestine regarded sickness and death as evil—a view embraced in our culture. As the natural human tendency is to resist death and disease, the master's recommendation would no doubt have been as unexpected then as it would be in this day and age. There was nevertheless a consistency in his approach as he also recommended that people "love their enemies."[1]

Between these two great philosophers, approximately 200 BC, came the *Yoga Sutras*, attributed to Patanjali. This work forms the basis of the science of yoga. It may in fact be even older, as much of it is based on the Vedas and Upanishads, the sacred scriptures of the Hindus.

Fighting at the physical level

The yoga principle "what you resist persists" can be demonstrated quite well in the area of competition. Our Western culture values competition not only in sport but also in economics and politics, where it forms the basis of our democratic, capitalist system. In business and politics, competition promotes efficiency and growth. It produces a similar situation in sport. If a young man wants to improve his tennis skills, he would be advised to compete against players more skilled than him. When an accomplished opponent attacks him with blistering serves and leaves him with stretching backhand returns, the young aspirant will either give up the game in frustration or become more proficient in the weaker areas of his game. Strong competition pinpoints weaknesses, inviting a dedicated player to work hard to overcome them. In other words, good opposition makes a competitor stronger.

Germ warfare is an example of this principle applied to the health scene. Doctors fight pathogenic bacteria with antibiotics and successfully eliminate them from patients' bodies. However, the bacteria as a species produce mutations, thereby breeding a new race of germs with the capacity to overcome the antibiotics. These mutated germs are a much stronger bunch of opponents than their forebears. The species appear to be flourishing on the battlefield of competition. So while physicians are winning the individual battles, they may be losing the war.

A similar picture emerges with cancer therapy. The initial treatment with chemotherapy or radiation usually produces a successful reduction in the size of the tumour. Unfortunately, subsequent courses of radiotherapy or chemotherapy provide diminishing returns as cancer cells become stronger in their capacity to withstand the barrage.

Fighting at the mental level

This same principle can be seen just as clearly at the mental level where fighting negative thoughts is so counterproductive. On the tennis court, I would angrily tell myself not to serve another double fault. One of my great friends who loves a little gamesmanship would remind me as I was about to tee off at golf not to think about the hazards near the tee. He knew the mind did not recognise the word 'not.' My subconscious seems to hear only the words 'double fault' and "drive your ball into the lake." Double faults and skewed drives have both been plentiful in my sporting life.

There was an amusing example of this principle in the television series *Faulty Towers*. German tourists were coming to stay at the hotel. Basil was running around telling the staff and long-term residents "not to talk about the war." Before long, he was goose-stepping with his finger over his lip, doing an impersonation of Hitler.

I had a ten-year battle with the 'yips,' an embarrassing problem for anyone trying to play golf. Standing over a short putt, my body would be a mass of moving parts. The ball could head in any direction

THE EAGLE'S WAY

off the putter, and it would frequently finish up farther away from the hole than where it had started. The more I tried to 'beat it,' the worse it got. If it were not for the social pleasures of the nineteenth hole, I would have given up the game. The problem started to resolve itself only when I stopped fighting it. I started to laugh at myself and stopped focusing on my score and on not yipping. Only as I detached from the need to be good at the game—to stop seeing it as though my self-worth depended on the scorecard—did the problem resolve.

In short, fighting negative thoughts serves only to keep them in mind, making it more likely the negative experience will persist.

Fighting at the verbal level

We can also get some idea of the problem at the verbal level. When people's behaviour is causing a problem, one may have an irresistible urge to shout at them to "stop it!" preferably "this instant." However, unless the recipient of this order is suitably fearful of the commander, this sort of demand will be met with opposition. It may come in the form of an angry response or a two-fingered salute, together with resistance in the form of continuation of the behaviour. Alternatively, it may be met with begrudging obedience but an underlying attitude of passive resistance. Such obedience may be followed by a determination to sabotage those orders at the earliest opportunity! Newton's second law of motion comes to mind: "To every action, there is an equal and opposite reaction."

As a culture, we have recognized the wisdom of not fighting unwanted habits. Psychologists generally recommend that parents do not focus on their children's unsavoury habits, such as picking their noses or playing with their genitals. Ignoring them may look like avoiding the issue, but at least it is starving the habits of attention. Prohibiting these habits draws attention to them, keeps them in mind, and helps them persist—albeit out of sight of the commander.

This may be part of the problem with making war on global undesirables. The wars on cancer, poverty, and terror have not produced any great returns. By keeping the focus on what we do *not* want, we may be getting more of the same.

DR. PETER L. JOHNSTON

Here in Victoria, the state government was concerned by the high cost of worker's compensation in the early 1990s. The major illness responsible was *repetitive strain injury*, known as RSI. It affected people doing any repetitive work, including data entry on computers. So the government in concert with the medical profession sent a letter to all doctors requesting the term RSI not be used. Doctors were asked to use specific terms like *tenosynovitis* for the same condition and apply it to each region of the body. Despite the simplicity of the campaign, it was remarkably successful in reducing the number of these complaints.

Fighting at the emotional level

Fighting negative emotions like sadness, grief, anger, guilt, and depression does not make them disappear. Negative emotions may successfully be held at bay for a time but not indefinitely. Holding off grief until after a funeral allows the aggrieved to mourn privately. Shelving anger until one can thrash the stuffing out of a pillow reduces the risk of spraying the anger all over one's spouse or an innocent bystander. Nevertheless, the popularity of emotional release workshops is founded on the value of allowing emotions to be expressed in a safe way rather than risk having them emerge in embarrassing or dangerous ways.

Fighting at the intuitive level

Fighting does not work at the intuitive level either. By intuition, I am referring to a 'sixth sense' that guides people. It is sometimes spoken of as the '*still, small voice*,' but it rarely manifests as an audible voice. More often it is an idea, a feeling, or just 'inner knowing.'

It may come as a 'gut reaction' letting us know that something is amiss—danger is at hand or someone is not telling us the truth. A more positive intuitive message is an urge towards something one's heart desires, be it a career, a hobby, a relationship, or something more trivial. This inner urge will frequently come from left field in the sense that it may be unexpected or unconventional. It may also be scary, as following one's intuition may not please others. One's family and culture generally prefer conformity and predictability.

The voice of intuition is indeed a small voice in the sense that it never insists or pushes, but it does not go away either. Fighting it does not work. Intuition derives from a deeper place I call the *soul*. The soul is another word for *psyche*. In Jungian terms, the psyche includes the personal and collective unconscious. These realms of consciousness contain knowledge far in excess of anything the conscious mind can ever know. They will be discussed in more depth in chapter seven.

Resisting an intuitive message may be blocking a soul destiny and can be costly. Life appears to have a way of encouraging people to take their destined paths. If one ignores the subtle whispers, dreams will tend to bring the same message in a coded but attention-seeking form. If the inner messages are still being ignored, outer messages may start arriving. They may come from books, the Internet, television, or comments from a friend. Ultimately, if nothing is attracting the desired attention, the message may hit in a more drastic form. It might take the form of bankruptcy, relationship breakdown, accident, or illness. Some writers in the New Age movement refer to such crises as 'wake-up calls.'

Fighting at the metaphorical level

It is interesting to look at the dominant metaphors we use in relation to good and evil. Angels and saintly figures are usually depicted in white robes with white wings or white lilies or with a halo of light around their heads. We use light to signify knowledge and wisdom too. We 'shed light' on a subject.

Conversely, evil characters are frequently shown in black. We speak of them as shady or dark characters. Sometimes they are obliging enough to wear that colour themselves. Hitler's Gestapo and many of the mafia are examples of this. We also describe ignorance as "being in the dark." The metaphor of the storm gains much of its force from the darkness that accompanies it. So we speak of black days, dark or even black moods, and dark times. Storms, like all dark moments of life may produce positive outcomes but these are spoken of as 'silver linings' to the dark clouds—and silver is a shining variety of white.

When white light is refracted through a pyramid-shaped lens, it breaks up into the colours of the spectrum. From these seven basic colours, blending can create all the other known shades—except black. So it could be said that white contains all colours. Hence, white is a symbol of wholeness as well as purity. Black, on the other hand, could be described as the absence of colour. Evil acts are done without any serious concern for the good of the whole. Given that they rebound on the perpetrator, such acts are also lacking in light and wisdom.

It does not make much sense to fight darkness, which is really an absence of light. The French and Russian revolutionaries fought against the darkness of their respective dysfunctional monarchies. When they succeeded in overthrowing those regimes, they replaced them with reigns of terror even darker than the regimes they had displaced.

What is needed is light. Once light shines in darkness, the darkness disappears. The philosophers quoted in this chapter shone light into an area of darkness. In doing so, they helped clear the darkness of ignorance with the light of wisdom.

C. The Practical Problems of Fighting

Because the majority of people attend their doctors for the purpose of finding some relief from their problems and discomfort, the conventional medical system works well. Like birds fighting against a storm, patients make considerable headway against their afflictions. However, as with the birds, they can also get knocked around a bit.

Side effects of medication

Many drugs aim at intervening in biochemical pathways but such interventions run into problems because the human body is so complex. Biochemical substances like hormones and neurotransmitters not only have multiple functions but can operate in totally different ways in different organs. So it is not surprising that most medications

THE EAGLE'S WAY

come with a lengthy list of potential side-effects relating to multiple organs and systems.

It had long been known that female sex hormones affected other organs but early research on hormone replacement therapy (HRT) suggested this treatment protected women against heart disease. In general, doctors were encouraged to recommend HRT to menopausal patients, not just to manage menopausal symptoms but to prevent osteoporosis and cardiovascular disease. The US National Institute of Health conducted a women's health initiative trial to assess the degree to which HRT was cardio-protective. The trial was abruptly stopped in July 2002 when it was found that women on HRT were at increased risk of heart attack, stroke, and breast cancer. While HRT medication is still available, sales plummeted after the publication of the trial.[2]

Non-steroidal anti-inflammatory agents (NSAIDs) are a large group of medications used for arthritis and musculoskeletal conditions. The best-known NSAIDs are aspirin and ibuprofen, both of which are available without a prescription in Australia. The problem with this group of drugs is that they all negatively impact the gastrointestinal system. They can cause indigestion and may trigger peptic ulceration. Bleeding from these peptic ulcers is not an infrequent cause of death in the elderly, and the elderly are the people most commonly suffering from arthritis. The more effective the NSAIDs are in helping arthritis pain, the more likely they are to cause side effects.[3]

Hence, the arrival of a new group of NSAID drugs called COX-2 inhibitors was greeted with enthusiasm as they had been found in trials to be less harsh on the stomach and duodenum. However, a later clinical study showed that there was an increased risk of heart attack and stroke beginning after eighteen months of treatment with Vioxx, one of the COX-2 inhibitors. In October 2004, the manufacturers issued a recall notice, and the drug was removed from the market in Australia.

The story of thalidomide is a salutary one. Marketed in the late 1950s, it was used as a sleeping pill and as a treatment for morning sickness in pregnancy. Grunenthal, a German pharmaceutical company, sold the drug in Germany, Britain, and about fifty other countries, including Australia. In 1961, scientists discovered the

DR. PETER L. JOHNSTON

medication stunted the growth of foetal arms and legs. Even one dose in early pregnancy was capable of severely affecting the growth of limbs. There were also reports of eye and ear defects and severe internal defects of heart, kidneys, and digestive and nervous systems. Worldwide, about twelve thousand babies were born with birth defects. In round figures, eight thousand survived their first year of life, nearly all surviving with their deformities.

The legacy of thalidomide has been extreme care in the use of drugs in the first three months of pregnancy. There have been no formal trials of any drug in pregnancy, so no medication is recommended for use in the first three months of pregnancy unless it has proved itself a safe drug prior to 1961.[4]

In most cases, ceasing medication will stop side effects. However, there are some serious side effects, such as bone marrow depression, which can be fatal. There are also a number of drugs capable of causing permanent damage to the eighth cranial nerve resulting in deafness.

Toxic effects of medications

All pharmaceutical products have an ideal dosage range that acts as a guideline for prescribing. Yet individuals vary so much in what they can tolerate. A sensitive person may require only 10 per cent of what another person of the same height and weight may need. If patients have any problems with kidney function, they will not be able to excrete the drug in the normal way, so a small dose may accumulate in the body. In either of these situations, a dose within the normal recommended range can be toxic to the recipient.

Toxic effects are also more likely with combined drugs. When the patients are elderly, especially if they have deteriorating memory and dementia, the incidence of accidental overdosing and toxic effects make the situation considerably more dangerous.

Some drugs are toxic by design. Most anti-cancer drugs are chosen because of their capacity to kill malignant cells. This is their modus operandi. The fact they are toxic to many normal cells comes under the heading of collateral damage. Ralph Moss, who has spent most of

THE EAGLE'S WAY

his life researching cancer therapies, believes chemotherapeutic drugs reduce the quality of a patient's life even more than their cancer does.[5]

Complications of surgery

The training and skill of surgeons in the Western world is generally of high quality. Nevertheless, even with good technique, competent surgeons, anaesthetists, and theatre staff, there are still significant risks associated with surgery. Bleeding can occur despite adequate haemostasis. Deep vein thrombosis and its potentially fatal complication, namely pulmonary embolus, can occur as a result of long operations and bed rest. Pneumonia is always a risk in the elderly, and wound infection can complicate any surgical procedure. These risks escalate with increasing age and level of illness prior to surgery.

Increasing resistance of microbes to drugs

A widespread problem is increasing drug resistance, especially in hospitals. It started with penicillin, but now some of these powerful, hospital-based germs, especially the golden staphylococcus, have become resistant to every known antibiotic. Because infections are not uncommon after surgery, having this type of bacteria in hospitals greatly increases the risk of death from otherwise treatable infections.

Unfortunately, bacteria seem to be developing resistance to antibiotics faster than new antibiotics can be developed. Resistance to medication is not limited to bacteria. The malarial parasite is outstripping efforts to control it with antimalarial drugs. As malaria is the commonest disease worldwide, this represents a serious problem.

Health costs in the medical system

The extent to which people are battered by the conflict between disease and its treatments is hard to gauge accurately. Lazarou and his associates reviewed thirty-nine prospective studies from hospitals in the United States between 1996 and 1999 and found serious adverse

DR. PETER L. JOHNSTON

reactions to medication in 6.7 per cent of all hospitalised patients, of which 0.32 per cent were fatal.[6]

Another study that also took into account hospital infections, surgical complications, and human error estimated 225,000 deaths annually in US hospitals. On these figures, death from iatrogenic causes would constitute the third largest cause of death in the United States, trailing only heart disease and cancer.[7]

To put this in perspective, the mortality and morbidity rate would be much greater if no treatment was instituted. Over 90 per cent of patients benefit from their hospitalisation. Nevertheless, the extent of complications is a cause for concern.

The financial costs of the system

With every advance in diagnostic technology and treatment, the cost of the medical system increases. Everywhere in the Western world, the financial burden is being felt. In Australia, hospitals have long waiting lists, and many of the public hospital wards are closed. There is constant pressure to discharge people from hospital and get them back home as quickly as possible.

With doctors and hospitals being held responsible for patient welfare, legal suits for negligence are becoming more common. Since UMP, the largest Australian medical indemnity insurance company, collapsed in 2002, the federal government has had to take steps to prop up the industry.[8]

For the parents of a child born with cerebral palsy, the financial burden is a heavy addition to the physical and emotional load they have to carry. The support they get from government sources is relatively small. It makes good sense for parents to sue the doctor and hospital for negligence, regardless of whether there are adequate grounds to claim negligence, especially when lawyers carry the cost of an unsuccessful suit. With sympathetic juries and doctors keen to avoid publicity, large awards have resulted. While this has been a positive result for the families involved, the hospitals and medical indemnity funds have been obliged to carry the cost. Such cases have caused the closure of country hospitals in Australia. It has also driven up the cost of medical indemnity insurance for midwifery to a level that the average family doctor cannot afford. Currently, less than 7 per cent of family doctors deliver babies.[9] This situation is creating problems for pregnant women in rural areas.

The human costs of the system

Large public hospitals are becoming more dangerous and unhealthy with more electromagnetic equipment, radioactive material, and multi-resistant microorganisms. They are also becoming more emotionally cold toward patients as it is harder to get attention from busy staff.

For nurses, the task of working faster to cover staff shortages, the increasing paperwork, and the lack of meaningful contact with patients all result in frustration and burn out for many.

In Australia, we have an acute shortage of nurses despite increases in the number of student places at tertiary institutions. The shortage seems to be due to a large number of qualified nurses ceasing to practise nursing. The traditional reason for withdrawing from the workforce to have a family is one factor. However, many are also working or studying complementary medicine, and others are in non-health-related jobs. The message I frequently hear from nurses is that they are leaving a health system in which they feel exploited. They are favouring work that values the nurturing and caring qualities that attracted them to nursing in the first place.

A survey in 1998 concluded that 53 per cent of Australian general practitioners had considered leaving general practice because of work stress.[10] Other statistics have suggested medicine to be an unhealthy way of life with doctors ahead of the general population in the figures for alcoholism, drug addiction, and suicide.[11] Male medical practitioners appear to be twice as likely to commit suicide as other professional males, while female practitioners are four to six times more likely to suicide than other professional women.[12]

DR. PETER L. JOHNSTON

Lack of patient empowerment

Many people take their bodies to their doctors in the same way they take their cars to their mechanics. There is hope and expectation that the doctor can find the cause of the problem and fix it. The underlying principle for both the doctor and the motor mechanic is that they are held responsible for "fixing the problem." Once clients give their cars to their mechanics, they usually relinquish all responsibility for the outcome—other than the responsibility to pay an appropriate fee. When they visit a doctor in Australia, they do not even need to do this if they hold a health-care card. In my previous clinic, 65 per cent of the patients paid no out-of-pocket expenses at all.

This lack of accountability for one's own health is a form of disempowerment. If health is dependent on the quality and quantity of foods and fluids ingested, air inhaled, emotions expressed or suppressed, physical exercise performed, and philosophies espoused and lived, then it is hard to see how anyone can ever truly hand over this responsibility to anyone else.

This responsibility issue has other costs too. While the onus is seen to be placed on the health practitioner rather than the individual, it creates an environment ideal for ambulance chasers. A case here in Australia in the late 1990s resulted in damages being awarded against a family doctor for not ensuring his patient actually attended the specialist to whom he referred her.[13]

CHAPTER 4

Avoiding The Storm

In general, birds have the strength and resources to handle brief storms. The brief storms in medicine are called acute illnesses. Examples are convulsions, abscesses, acute abdomens, viral infections, and attacks of migraine and asthma. Serious acute infections like meningitis and pneumonia can be handled capably by conventional medicine. Acute, life-threatening medical, surgical, and obstetrical emergencies, including cardiac arrests, can be overcome. It is this area of acute and dramatic illness that represents the pinnacle of triumph for twentieth-century medicine.

The problem occurs when a storm rages on and the resources of the bird are stretched. A bird that has tried to overcome the storm but found the task too demanding will tend to head for a safe haven. In a similar fashion, the doctor faced with a problem for which his training and knowledge has no ready answers tends to head for the safety of symptom relief. Symptom relief is very important to both patient and doctor but it is not curing the disease.

Avoidance in Mainstream Medicine

The medical storm that rages on is called *chronic disease.* Doctors are not the only people who struggle with chronic disease. Most can handle short-lived problems, but prolonged illness tends to drain

DR. PETER L. JOHNSTON

the resources of not only the patient and the doctor but also the family and carers. Chronic disease can be divided into a number of categories.

1. Congenital and hereditary disease

Congenital abnormalities vary from minor structural deficiencies to severe malformations incompatible with life. At this time, surgery is the most effective treatment for conditions like harelip and cleft palate. As surgical technology has advanced, previously incurable congenital conditions have become amenable to surgery. Serious heart abnormalities are routinely repaired, and successful attempts have been made to separate Siamese twins.

Prevention consists mainly of screening the newborn for inborn metabolic diseases like phenylketonuria and screening potential parents for the presence of genes predisposing their children to congenital abnormalities. When the parental genetic configuration shows a serious risk of having children with debilitating, life-threatening diseases like haemophilia or Huntington's chorea, the recommended course of action is to avoid a conventional pregnancy. Techniques for in vitro fertilization using donor cells avoid the transmission of the abnormal genes.

It has long been assumed that congenital diseases derive from inheriting a faulty gene from one or other parent. There are about 26,000 genes laid out in human DNA. When research began on the human genome project, there was much optimism that genetic manipulation might provide cures. One of the first diseases studied was sickle cell anaemia caused by a single gene defect. However, the common diseases turned out to be much more complex. High blood pressure and diabetes involve sixty or more genes, making intervention very difficult.

A further complication was the discovery of proteins surrounding the DNA, which not only affected the manifestation of genetic material but could also be transmitted to later generations. The study of this matter is called 'epigenetics'. This is now the more promising area of research because it is where environmental factors can have their influence. As an example, my wife and her two sisters inherited a genetic disorder called alpha-1-antitrypsin deficiency. All three were nurses and they all smoked. The combination of the missing enzyme and smoking led to emphysema in all three. However while one died at forty, the other two have reached mid-sixties, albeit disabled. Although they all had the genetic defect, they might have led normal lives if they had never smoked. Presumably other epigenetic factors have dictated their different outcomes. Epigenetics is showing us that both nature and nurture are involved in hereditary disease and environmental factors can be changed.

2. Traumatic disease

Trauma can also produce chronic disability. Motor vehicle accidents and sports injuries can damage any part of the body, ranging from a crushed little toe to quadriplegia. Injuries can also lead to chronic disease. Severe or recurrent knee injuries can lead to chronic arthritis in later life. Multiple head injuries from boxing can lead to Parkinson's disease or dementia.

Injuries are not categorised as chronic diseases in themselves but are contributing factors to the development of chronic disease.

3. Deficiency diseases

There are two main areas of deficiency that can result in disease.

a) Vitamin and mineral deficiency

The major problem with chronic diseases is the lack of available cures. Vitamin deficiencies are the exception. James Lind, a British Naval surgeon, wrote his famous *Treatise on Scurvy* in 1754, a book in which he stressed the need for citrus fruits on board ships. At that time, the navy was losing more men to scurvy than to combat. Maybe he forgot to write 'priority' on it, because it took another forty years for the British Navy to act on his recommendations. Once implemented, the disease virtually disappeared.[1]

DR. PETER L. JOHNSTON

Not until the twentieth century were vitamins clearly identified as the missing ingredients in scurvy and beriberi. In 1906, Sir Frederick Hopkins, a British biochemist, demonstrated that foods contained necessary 'accessory factors' in addition to proteins, carbohydrates, fats, minerals, and water. In 1912, Casimir Funk identified the missing ingredient in polished rice to be an amine. So he called it a *vital amine*, a term that eventually embraced all the 'accessory factors' and was abbreviated to *vitamins*. The discovery of a whole range of vitamins is one of the significant achievements of the twentieth century.[2]

Except for vitamin D, all vitamins are provided in food. Deficiencies occur in the Western world when diets are inadequate. This occurs mainly in alcoholics, elderly people living alone, and those with anorexia. They also occur when diets are adequate but a person's digestive system is unable to absorb the vitamins. Vitamin supplements given by injection can assist the latter.

The major region of vitamin deficiency is the Third World, where the lack of vitamins forms part of an overall state of malnutrition. There is an unequal distribution despite there being ample food on this planet to feed everyone. The problem is being avoided at the political and economic level, and resolution will require a global response. (On a positive note, in 2005, steps were taken to deal with poverty in Africa, the poorest continent on the globe.)

Mineral deficiencies are found in a number of chronic conditions. Their importance is being increasingly recognised in the Western world with the move toward more processed foods in the diet. If the diet is deficient, minerals can nearly all be given as oral supplements, either in a celloid or chelated form.

The treatment of vitamin and mineral deficiencies with dietary modifications or supplements fulfils my criteria for 'eagle's way medicine.' Vitamin and mineral supplements are not about fighting disease or avoiding it. The supplements provide something the body is missing. They contribute to the person becoming more whole.

THE EAGLE'S WAY

b) Hormone deficiencies

The discovery of insulin in 1921 by Banting and Best marked a turning point for diabetics, providing a significant extension of life expectancy for diabetics. In the pre-insulin days, juvenile diabetics died at an early age from ketosis.

Hormones from the thyroid, adrenal, parathyroid, and pituitary glands also came into use in the twentieth century—as did sex hormones. Unlike vitamins and minerals, hormones do not come from outside the body. The endocrine glands produce them naturally, and their level of production is controlled by a feedback system under the control of the pituitary gland.

If a natural or synthetic hormone is administered, the pituitary gland detects its presence, and if it assesses the new hormone level as adequate, the pituitary gland will not produce any of its own stimulating hormones. This is the *modus operandi* of the contraceptive pill. Administering hormones discourages endocrine glands from producing their own natural hormones, so ovulation does not occur.

Once a vital gland is no longer functioning either through disease, removal, or suppression, a constant lifelong supply of replacement hormone is required. Hence, patients with diabetes, hypothyroidism, adrenal failure (Addison's disease), and hypopituitarism require long-term management.

This 'management' is life-saving and compassionate but should not be confused with healing or curing. Hormone replacement is not bringing the glands back into function. In fact, it may be suppressing any residual glandular function. At this time, medical science has not discovered how to facilitate glandular function. What hormone replacement does is reduce the symptoms of the disease and allow the patient to survive.

Hence, management with hormone replacement, while extremely important, is not unlike the birds avoiding the storm. It provides safety, survival and comfort but makes no real progress against the storm, which continues unabated. If the management of a patient with diabetes is thorough and their blood sugars remain stable, the patient should be symptom-free. However, the disease is not really being addressed.

DR. PETER L. JOHNSTON

Management with diet, drugs, and insulin is not always going to prevent the later complications of the disease that tend to manifest in the small blood vessels of the kidneys, eyes, and legs.

4. Chronic inflammation

Acute inflammations could be compared to full-scale wars in which the body's defence system mobilises all its resources against an invader. An invasion of the lungs by bacteria can result in pneumonia. In the pre-antibiotic era, pneumonia was truly a fight to the death—a fight culminating in a crisis. The patient would either die or fully recover. Either way, the bacteria would die, theirs being a kamikaze mission.

Chronic inflammations, comparatively speaking, are more like long, drawn-out border disputes. They simmer on with sporadic outbursts of fighting with no clear victory. The battleground meanwhile becomes more damaged and less supportive of life. The patient lives on, but the quality of life diminishes.

The common chronic infections of the nineteenth century were tuberculosis and syphilis. These were both caused by bacteria, which at least provided an enemy to fight. Antibiotics made big inroads against these old enemies, so much so that they now play relatively minor roles in the developed nations. The major microbial enemy is now the AIDS virus, against which medical science has developed weapons in the form of antiviral medications.

Nowadays, most of the other chronic inflammations have no identified pathogen, and we are left with a battle against an invisible foe. Examples of these are the following:

- Chronic glomerulonephritis: inflammation of the kidneys
- Chronic pancreatitis: inflammation of the pancreas
- Ulcerative colitis: inflammation of the large bowel
- Chronic hepatitis: inflammation of the liver
- Rheumatoid arthritis: inflammation of the joints
- Thyroiditis: inflammation of the thyroid gland

THE EAGLE'S WAY

5. Degenerative disease

This large group of diseases represents conditions that tend to occur in old age but can also occur earlier. The brain and nervous system are affected by the hardening of the arteries, which, along with Alzheimer's disease, can gradually progress to a serious level of dementia, or it can erupt suddenly with a stroke that can paralyse an arm and leg and affect one's capacity for expression through speech, facial movements, and writing. Parkinson's disease and motor neuron disease both affect mobility and impair the bodily expression of emotions.

The sense organs also degenerate. Hearing is commonly impaired in the elderly, starting with the high-frequency sounds. In the eyes, lenses harden, and by the age of fifty, most Westerners are using reading glasses to compensate for long-sightedness. Later, the lenses become cloudy, a condition known as cataracts, for which surgery can work wonders. Unfortunately, when the retina degenerates (a condition called macular degeneration), there are no magic cures, and the patients lose their vision.

The genital organs also degenerate. In males, the prostate gland tends to enlarge, and the sperm count declines in both number and mobility. In females, the vagina tends to atrophy and become dry.

Bones become brittle with osteoporosis, while joints can become more rigid and painful with arthritis. Almost any organ of the body can be affected by arteriosclerosis, a hardening of the arteries feeding those organs.

Cirrhosis of the liver is a degenerative disease that tends to occur earlier in life but mainly as a complication of alcoholism or hepatitis.

Calculi, especially gallstones and kidney stones, while degenerative in nature, occur at younger ages.

6. Hyperplastic disease

Hyperplasia is an increased rate of the reproduction of cells, creating an enlarged organ. Unlike tumours, the enlargement is more orderly. However, it occurs mainly in glandular organs, so it can result in excess production of hormones. Surgery can be helpful but rarely curative.

DR. PETER L. JOHNSTON

7. Neoplastic disease

Neoplastic is the medical term used to describe all growths and tumours. Malignant growths in organs are called carcinomas. In skeletal tissues, these are called sarcomas, and in blood, these are called leukaemias. Finally, in lymph tissue, these are called lymphomas. Grouped under the banner of *cancer*, they represent the second largest cause of death in the Western world.

While cancer occurs in every age group, even infants, it is more common in the older age groups. When the disease spreads, it invades organs and tissues. It interferes with the cells and the blood supply to the organ, resulting in degeneration of that organ—and ultimately the whole body. The body's defence system does resist the onslaught, but there is far less evidence of resistance than there is in chronic inflammation.

When cancer has spread beyond its site of origin, it is referred to as metastatic or secondary cancer. At this level, it acts like a degenerative disease, producing wasting. Current thinking on the causes of cancer suggest the body produces mutated cells quite frequently, but the killer T-cells of the body's defence system eliminate them. Electron microscope photographs of killer cells destroying a cancer cell can be seen on the website for immunotherapy.[3] It is when the body's defence system is rundown that cancer can get a hold. The immune system tends to degenerate with age, so in some ways, cancer is a degenerative disease of the immune system.

Cancer differs from the other degenerative diseases in having a visible enemy. However, unlike infection, where the enemy is an invader from outside, cancer attacks from within. A cancer cell changes from a normal, cooperative, and disciplined cell into a wild, selfish, aggressive, destructive cell. Unlike antibiotics, our weapons against these invaders are not as discerning. Chemotherapy and radiotherapy do not clearly differentiate between cancer cells and other young, immature cells. Because of this lack of specificity in treatment, it is not possible to kill off all the metastatic cancer cells around the body without fatally damaging cells in the blood and bone marrow. For this reason, the treatment is referred to as palliative, not curative. Its goal is to prolong life, not to eradicate the disease. So in a sense, it is fighting two enemies—disease and death.

Management of chronic disease

A clear understanding of the cause of chronic disease is lacking. Because one expects to grow old and die, it is also expected that body parts will degenerate—a process called *entropy*. However, entropy does not entirely explain why one person's physical and mental functioning is sharp and agile at one hundred years of age while another person has Alzheimer's disease at sixty.

Unless chronic inflammation is caused by microorganisms, such as tubercle bacilli in TB or tropical parasites in malaria and bilharzia, there are no enemies to fight. Without an understanding of the causes of these diseases, we have no weapons with which to fight the process. Conventional management techniques of chronic disease are as follows:

- Pain relief with analgesics or anti-inflammatory agents. For more severe chronic pain, relief may be achieved by severing the nerve transmitting the pain.
- Relief of other symptoms like nausea and diarrhoea with medication.
- Suppression of the body's defence system in chronic inflammation by using corticosteroids. It is akin to reducing the casualties of war by withdrawing some of one's own troops. Nevertheless, it usually produces rapid relief of the symptoms.
- Compensation for diminished function as in using spectacles for presbyopia, the long-sightedness of middle age.
- Replacement of the function of the diseased organ by using pancreatic enzymes in chronic pancreatitis or by using dialysis (artificial kidney) in chronic nephritis.
- Removal of the inflamed organ or part thereof, the lining of large arteries for arteriosclerosis, or sections of bowel in ulcerative colitis and Crohn's disease.

DR. PETER L. JOHNSTON

- Replacement of damaged organs with transplants (e.g. the liver and kidney).
- Replacement of grossly affected joints with mechanical prostheses.
- The use of palliative care, mainly in cancer.

Like the bird finding shelter from the storm, this management makes the patient as safe and comfortable as possible while the war within continues unabated. The underlying disease process is really not being addressed. Although it is not openly acknowledged, the diseases are assumed to be incurable. Therefore, the issue of cure is avoided.

The problem of masking

One of the basic rules we learned in medical school was never to give strong pain relief to somebody with acute abdominal pain until we had a clear idea of the cause of the pain. The 'acute abdomen' is a surgical emergency that could be caused by a wide range of conditions. Among the potential diagnoses are appendicitis, pancreatitis, gallstones, stone in the ureter, perforated peptic ulcer, ruptured ectopic pregnancy, Crohn's disease, ruptured ovarian cysts, or diverticulae.

Any ruptured organ can be fatal without emergency surgery. On the other hand, Crohn's disease and pancreatitis are aggravated by surgery. Abdominal pain is understood as a message from the body, letting the patient and doctor know that something is amiss. By examining the patient while the pain is still giving off its signal, the doctor is able to feel tenderness in certain areas and detect signs to help diagnose the problem.

If, however, narcotics are administered to patients prior to their being seen by the doctor, the pain is suppressed, and with it, some of the vital clues to diagnosis are masked. A leaking appendix might quietly progress to a life-threatening peritonitis without the telltale signals that would otherwise alert the surgeon. Suppression of symptoms is called '*masking*.' The giving of narcotic pain relief to patients with acute abdominal pain is akin to silencing the messenger rather than listening to the message. The symptom is like the warning light

THE EAGLE'S WAY

on the dashboard of the car. Relieving the symptom without addressing the cause is like removing the fuse to stop the light flashing.

From a similar perspective, the medical treatment of chronic disease could be viewed as 'masking.' When one is purely treating the symptoms rather than the cause, the message from the body is silenced. The body may be trying to alert us to the fact there is something amiss. The warning light is not being acted upon because it is being turned off.

Provided that there is awareness of this, there is no problem. Adequate relief from pain and nausea is very important, necessary, and humane, but the ideal is for patients to seek the cause of their problem while they get adequate symptom relief at the same time.

Avoidance in Mainstream Psychiatry

The American Psychiatric Association has produced a classification of mental disease in a large book called the DSM-III. With the exception of organic psychoses, such as dementia and delirium, where pathological changes can be found in the brain, there are no physical abnormalities to be found in mental disease. Psychiatry deals with mental and emotional problems and their manifestations in abnormal behaviour.

Clinical psychology also deals with these same problems. There are many different theories and models of psychology that can guide different practitioners of either modality. There is one major difference between psychiatrists and psychologists. Namely, psychiatrists have medical degrees and can legally prescribe medication to a client. Drug treatment is, in fact, the main therapy used to manage psychiatric disorders in mainstream psychiatry, albeit in conjunction with various forms of counselling.

With little in the way of physical signs other than abnormal behaviour, the diagnosis of mental disease rests mainly on the history given by the patients and their relatives. Diagnosis in psychiatry is not only bereft of organic changes but also has less clear diagnostic syndromes than physical medicine. Most psychiatric diagnoses are descriptions of emotional states like depression, anxiety, hyperactivity, mania, schizophrenia (translated as split personality), and obsessive-compulsion. Much importance is placed on diagnosing the dom-

DR. PETER L. JOHNSTON

inant state of mind. Yet this is very difficult because most patients present with a mixed picture. It is uncommon for patients to have a pure anxiety state without some depressive symptoms and vice versa.

It is unwise to give a depressed patient an anti-anxiety drug only, as the reduction in anxiety might give the patient the strength to commit suicide. Nevertheless, the main benefit in defining the major emotion involved is in making it easier to treat. If doctors diagnose an anxiety state, they can prescribe anti-anxiety drugs. If they diagnose depression, they can prescribe antidepressants. There are also drugs to treat obsessive-compulsive states and schizophrenia. To a lesser extent, this labelling happens in psychology as well. With so many schools of thought about how the psyche works, it gives a feeling of confidence to therapists if they can fit the client's symptom picture into a pattern they can understand and treat.

Avoidance in anxiety

It seems reasonable to assume that if people are anxious, there is some valid reason for this, be it conscious or unconscious. Drugs may reduce the impact of anxiety, but they are not dealing with the cause. It may be helpful, kind, and compassionate to administer medication to reduce anxiety, but if medication is the only treatment being instituted, the problem is being avoided.

The benzodiazepines are a group of drugs used for anxiety and insomnia, a group that includes Valium, Serepax, Xanax and Mogadon. It took years to discover that using any of these drugs for four months or more could lead to addiction. Ceasing the drugs or even just staying on the same dose led to withdrawal effects. The chief symptom of withdrawal was anxiety. Because anxiety was the usual reason the drug was prescribed in the first place, doctors naturally assumed the patient's anxiety was due to the dose of medication being too low. So their tendency was to increase the dose, thereby compounding the addiction.

In the early 1980s, I prescribed a very small dose of Valium for a patient with blepharospasm, a painful twitching of the eyelids. She was a meditation teacher with no other evidence of anxiety. But

THE EAGLE'S WAY

after she was on the Valium for six months, she developed chronic anxiety. I started to increase the dose before I learned that anxiety could be caused by Valium. The next step involved a long period of withdrawal for her.

Even after full withdrawal, she never really regained her pre-treatment level of relaxation.

Once the addictive propensity of benzodiazepines was discovered, their use was quarantined. Nowadays, they are used mainly in short bursts for acute emotional crises and for muscle relaxation in acute pain states. Nevertheless, it remains a cautionary tale. Dealing with stress and anxiety by using 'quick fixes' in the form of medication, nicotine, alcohol or recreational drugs can bring a heavy cost. Farther down the path lies the problem of addiction with the initial problem remaining unresolved.

Like the birds seeking shelter from the storm, tranquillisers provide a temporary shelter and safe haven from overpowering emotions. However, staying in this safe haven is counterproductive if one is going to be dragged from the shelter by side effects and pushed into an even more treacherous storm.

Avoidance in depression

Depression is indeed a depressing condition. Like a drab, gray mantle over everything, sufferers can feel no joy, fun, or excitement in their lives. They often wake between two and four in the morning when anxious and depressing thoughts can run wild. Their appetites diminish. In many cases, their appetite for life diminishes to the point where they choose to end it.

Depressed patients are a serious concern to their doctors. As a family doctor, I always felt a sense of urgency about helping lift patients out of depression. This partially came from a sense of concern and compassion, but there was also a selfish aspect to it. The potential for suicide made it imperative for me to do something constructive. While I have not been compelled to answer difficult questions in a coroner's court, I have faced the sad task of trying to explain the suicide of a depressed patient to a bereaved family.

DR. PETER L. JOHNSTON

When the first group of antidepressant drugs, the tricyclics, came onto the market, it would be fair to say I grasped them enthusiastically, as did most of my medical colleagues. In the 1960s, we saw them as a major breakthrough because they were the first drugs to specifically target depression. In the 1970s and early 1980s, the main difference between the treatment of depression by general practitioners and that of psychiatrists was in the dosage of tricyclics. As a general practitioner, I prescribed no more than six amitriptyline tablets per day. If the patients were not responding, I would send them to psychiatrists who would prescribe up to twelve tablets per day.

The effectiveness of tricyclics helped confirm a theory about depression being a biochemical abnormality in the brain. The tricyclics had short-term unpleasant side effects, mainly dry mouth and blurred vision. However, over a longer term, weight gain proved a more problematical side effect. Six months of tricyclic treatment could leave some patients twenty kilograms heavier, giving them another reason to feel depressed. They were also effective as a means of suicidal overdose. As a result, the tricyclics now play a less prominent role in the treatment of depression.

In the late 1980s, the selective serotonin reuptake inhibitors, known as SSRIs, supplanted the tricyclics. Prozac, the first of the group, hit the market with a blaze of publicity, and in 2006, it had worldwide sales in excess of twenty billion dollars.

However, as usage has increased, the side effects have become more apparent, especially among the young. In 2004, the US Food and Drug Administration told the drug companies to harden their warnings about the potential side effects of SSRIs. They were compelled to include the words: "Antidepressants increase the risk of suicidal thinking and behaviour in children and adolescents with depression and other psychiatric disorders." The British National Health Service put it even more strongly. It advised doctors to stop prescribing SSRIs to patients younger than eighteen in the early stages of depression because of the link to suicidal thinking.[4]

The SSRIs are also coming under attack from other quarters. While Pfizer, the manufacturer of the popular SSRI called Zoloft, asserts that "SSRIs work by correcting the chemical imbalance in

THE EAGLE'S WAY

your brain," others are not so sure. Dr. Jon Jureidini, head of the department of psychological medicine at the Women's and Children's Hospital in Adelaide, put it this way:

> *The chemical imbalance theory is nonsense. SSRIs alter patients' serotonin levels within days, but their antidepressant effect—if there is any—does not occur for several weeks. The idea that there is a serotonin deficiency explaining depression is such a gross oversimplification as to be completely misleading. A lot of doctors and others are prone to wishful thinking.*[5]

On reviewing clinical trials, some researchers have concluded that SSRIs are scarcely more effective than placebo in alleviating depression. Dr. Joanna Moncrieff, senior lecturer in social and community psychiatry at the University College in London, has described SSRIs as "*more or less completely useless.*" Together with Irving Kirsch, professor of psychology at the University of Plymouth, they have stated, "*It is time for a thorough re-evaluation of current approaches to depression and further development of alternatives to drug treatment.*"[6]

In retrospect, it seems to me that our medical approach to depression has been Procrustean.[7] As doctors, we desperately wanted a treatment to alleviate depression, preferably a quick, easy, chemical solution. Necessity being the father of invention, the pharmaceutical companies provided what we needed. We did not want to look too closely at this gift. We wanted to make both the theory and the drugs fit the need. With the benefit of hindsight, perhaps the deeper problems of depression have been avoided.

Modern medicine and the soul

The words "psychology" and "psychiatry" both stem from the Greek word *psyche*, which means *soul*. Psychology translates as 'the study of the soul' and psychiatry as 'the treatment of the soul'. The soul is defined by the *Oxford Dictionary* as 'the spiritual or immaterial part of a human, regarded as immortal.' *Encyclopaedia Britannica* defines it as "the immaterial aspect or essence of a human being; that which confers individuality, which partakes of divinity and survives the death of the body."

These definitions create something of a contradiction, as mainstream teachings in psychology and psychiatry do not recognise the existence of the soul. The soul has religious overtones, which renders it unsuitable for scientific disciplines like medicine and psychology. Science also requires precise measurement, which the soul cannot provide. In fact, the soul cannot even be adequately observed. The soul in esoteric literature is frequently described as the *Self* (with a capital to differentiate it from the perceived 'self' of personality or ego. Frances Vaughan described the Self as being able to be experienced but not known as an object.[8] Her words are reminiscent of those of St. Francis of Assisi eight hundred years earlier: "*Perhaps what we seek is what is doing the seeking.*"

In defence of mainstream psychology and psychiatry, there are cogent historical reasons for this reluctance to admit metaphysical or religious concepts into their thinking. Scientific exploration had been stifled for nearly twelve hundred years, partly because of the control of an authoritarian church. The Christian church believed in the resurrection of the dead and saw the body as the "temple of the Holy Spirit." So dissection of cadavers was prohibited. Even when the church finally allowed the human body to be dissected, they held on to the right to administer to the soul while the doctors tended to the body. Only in the twentieth century, when growth in psychological knowledge was accompanied by a decline in the power and influence of the mainstream Christian churches, did the psychiatric and psychological disciplines take over the psyche. It is interesting that in our Western system, the separation of mind from body still continues. Psychiatrists do not like to have patients with physical problems in their hospital beds any more than physicians or surgeons like patients with psychiatric problems in their medical and surgical wards.

What the body-doctors and the mind-doctors do have in common, at least on the mainstream level, is a disinterest in anything that uses words like God, religion, or spiritual. They can hardly be blamed for their lack of enthusiasm for the spiritual. The separation of medicine from religion has helped produce the advanced system we now have. Why go backward into what they perceive to be a world of unproven dogma and superstition?

Yet in evicting the soul from mainstream psychiatry and medical science in general, I believe something extremely valuable has been lost. As Albert Einstein put it, *"Not everything that counts can be counted and not everything that can be counted counts."*[9]

Transpersonal experiences

Altered states of consciousness have been a part of indigenous cultural life since prehistoric times. Ceremonial dances and rituals, including breathing techniques, led people into trance states. Some cultures were aided in this process by the use of natural hallucinogenic substances, such as magic mushrooms and peyote.

Franz Mesmer, an Austrian physician, introduced hypnosis to Europe in the eighteenth century. However, it was the hippie culture of the 1960s with its widespread experimentation with hallucinogenic drugs that brought an understanding of altered states of consciousness to public awareness. Into the language of the Western world came the expressions 'other dimensions,' 'out-of-body experiences,' 'astral travelling,' 'near-death experiences,' and 'having a spiritual experience.' They all describe altered states of consciousness or transpersonal experiences.

In a similar way, I see mainstream psychology and psychiatry generally ignoring the widespread phenomenon of transcendental experiences. Out-of-body experiences do not sit easily with a philosophy equating the mind with the brain. If people are indeed comprised only of bodies controlled by brains, they should not be capable of seeing themselves outside their bodies.

Hallucinations

The materialistic approach to life also impacts the psychiatric attitude toward hallucinations. *Hallucination* is defined as the experience of perceiving objects or events not actually present to the senses. They are most commonly found in major psychotic states and conditions

DR. PETER L. JOHNSTON

like schizophrenia. Consequently, non-drug-induced hallucinations are viewed with concern as they might indicate the onset of psychosis.

Little wonder people have tended to be shy with regard to talking about such experiences. Medical authorities have the right to certify individuals and admit them to mental hospitals against their wills. If they are hallucinating and are diagnosed as schizophrenic, they may be considered incapable of making rational decisions for themselves. Hence, it may be deemed appropriate to hospitalise them for their own protection and for the protection of others. While it may well be the most appropriate course of action, the stakes are high for the patient in many cases. A diagnosis of schizophrenia can mean isolation from family and from all that is meaningful to the patient. Because the diagnosis can hinge on having hallucinations, it should be of paramount importance to have a clear idea of the nature of hallucination.

Yet this does not seem to be the case. In mainstream psychiatry, there appears to be no understanding that hallucinations could occur in a sane person. All hallucinations are seen as pathological. If a modern-day Francis of Assisi were to be brought to hospital by concerned relatives, he would have a strong chance of being institutionalised. Seeing visions and hearing voices have been the trademark of mystics throughout the ages, but there does not appear to be a place for these in our modern scientific system.

Of course, it makes diagnosis easier if all hallucinations are considered pathological. It means there is no need to assess the content, quality, and degree of integration of the hallucinatory material. Yet it is in the actual message of the hallucination that much can be gleaned, according to 'transpersonal psychiatrists.' To label an experience as a hallucination without exploring its meaning is not only avoiding the problem but might be creating a problem where none exists.

Dr. Stanislav Grof, the co-founder of the transpersonal psychology movement, warned against this:

> *What is normal and what is pathological should not be based on the content and nature of these experiences but on the way in which they are handled; on the degree to which a person can integrate these unusual experiences into his or her life. Harmonious integration*

of transpersonal experiences is crucial to mental health. Sympathetic support and assistance in this process is of critical importance to a successful therapy.[10]

To quote another pioneer of transpersonal psychology, Dr. R. D. Laing: "*The experiences of schizophrenics are often indistinguishable from those of mystics. Mystics and schizophrenics find themselves in the same ocean, but the mystics swim whereas the schizophrenics drown.*"[11]

In summary, the nature and complexity of hallucinations are avoided in mainstream medicine.

Synchronicity

Carl Jung was consulting with a female patient who had proved resistant to psychotherapy. She described a dream in which she had been presented with a golden scarab beetle. While he was analysing the dream, Jung heard a sound at the window. Lifting the sash, he found a rare scarab-like beetle on the sill trying to get inside. He picked up the beetle and showed it to his patient. This coincidence had a great impact on the patient. From that moment on, she made remarkable progress.[12] Jung saw and experienced many synchronicities that led him to write a famous work titled *Synchronicity: An Acausal Connecting Principle*. Although the word *synchronicity* is similar to the word *coincidence* in its definition, Jung actually coined the word to describe coincidences where meaningful external events occur in relation to internal psychic states.

Synchronicity has its theoretical base in Jung's concept of the *collective unconscious* and will be addressed in more detail in Chapter 10. While Jung remains an important figure in the history of modern psychology, his work finds few adherents in the mainstream. As a result, people who talk of coincidences are viewed with suspicion. After all, people who suffer from schizophrenia are prone to see meaning in events that have no logical connection at all.

DR. PETER L. JOHNSTON

The approach to death

When the scientific world view evicted the concept of the soul, it was left with no concept of self beyond the physical material world. Instead of an immortal soul that lived beyond the confines of time and space, there was only a body guided by a mind dwelling within the brain. Because the brain dies with the body, materialistic science sees death as the end of life.

No doubt this belief has been a driving force in producing our ingenious, life-saving technology. Paradoxically, it may also have been a motivating force to build up weapons of mass destruction. In the Second World War, the Japanese had trouble understanding the American approach to preserving lives. To a country encouraging kamikaze pilots, the tendency for US forces to use any amount of expensive military hardware rather than risk the lives of ground troops seemed strange. This cultural difference was still visible in the Iraq conflict. The leaders of the 'coalition of the willing' were keenly aware of the importance of minimising casualties among their troops. Meanwhile, in the extremist Arab world, suicide bombers seemed to be queuing up for service. When death equates to absolute annihilation, almost anything can be justified in preventing it.

Medical and surgical treatments involving hair loss and mutilation have all been pursued. I remember seeing a photograph in a surgery journal of a man who had had a surgical procedure for cancer. It was called a 'hemi-corporectomy.' The whole lower half of his body was removed, and he was pictured getting around on a flat trolley by paddling with his hands.

For all its wonderful technology and loving intent, it is hard to escape the feeling that the underlying motive for life-saving work has been fear. Not only is there a fight against death, but the whole subject of death has been avoided as being too negative to bear thinking about.

However, fear is an emotion with strong energy. It does not go away just because someone does not want to think about it. Repressing it just ensures it pops up whenever a trigger arises. People can tune out much of the death that surrounds them until someone

THE EAGLE'S WAY

close to them dies. Then emotions emerge and frequently swamp these individuals.

While free will is inherent, I believe everybody has a purpose in their life, whether they are conscious of it or not. Without it, they would have no basis for the choices they make. They would be like children in a supermarket, just grabbing whatever they could reach. The fact that people make choices means they do have some sort of value system—even if they cannot articulate it. Nevertheless, a value system ignoring something as inevitable as death has to be incomplete.

Dying may be physically painful and prolonged, or it might be sudden and unexpected with no time to say farewell to loved ones. It may interrupt one's life's work so the individual can go to realms unknown and unconsidered. It is hardly a scenario to relax into. It is no wonder terminal illness, death, bereavement, and grieving are such stressful times in our Western culture, both for the dying and their families.

Sadly, the physicians and psychiatrists who share this scientific world view are of limited help at these times. If they have not faced their own mortality, their own fears arise and can be felt by those they seek to comfort. When I worked in hospitals in the sixties, the dying patients were kept away from the rest of the patients in the public wards and were bypassed by the physicians on the ward rounds.

The work of Dr. Elisabeth Kubler-Ross in listening to dying patients brought a new understanding to the care of the dying. She was the first person to describe the stages of grief most patients endure in their last journey. Dying patients, before they can reach a stage of accepting their impending death, frequently experience denial, bargaining, anger, and depression.[13] The hospice movement evolved from Elisabeth's work. In hospices, the dying are nursed separately—in an environment more geared to caring for their physical and emotional needs. Most hospices do not cater to spiritual needs as such but allow and encourage patients to be visited by spiritual advisers of their own choice.

CHAPTER 5

The Art Of Medicine

The brief look at metaphysics in the previous chapter suggests conventional medical therapies are tending to ignore the inner origins of illness. They also involve fighting, which seems to contravene the advice of the masters of wisdom. Yet the effectiveness of mainstream medicine and surgery are beyond any doubt. I believe there are three reasons for this.

Firstly, while fighting problems may keep the problems in mind, a knockout punch is a different matter. It finishes the fight. Antibiotics knock out bacterial enemies. Removal of the appendix or gallbladder usually cures the pains associated with disease in these organs. Modern medicine is very effective in curing acute illness.

Secondly, the scientific validity of mainstream medicine is a source of its effectiveness, not only in acute illness but also in chronic conditions.

However, there is a third reason for the success of mainstream therapies. A look at the art of medicine rather than the science of medicine may shed some light on this healing factor.

In my search for knowledge about healing, my lower back pain has been a good teacher. For thirty years, I have had recurrent episodes of lumbar pain of varying severity, usually triggered by overwork, unscientific lifting, or hitting golf balls too aggressively. Over

THE EAGLE'S WAY

the years, I have experimented with a wide range of therapies—more out of convenience than because of dissatisfaction with any of them.

A family doctor, an osteopath, a few chiropractors, and a Japanese martial arts instructor have all had turns at manipulating my back. Quite dramatic relief followed each of these manoeuvres. Masseurs, kinesiologists, and Bowen therapists applied gentler techniques to my back, again successfully. More subtle was the work of a Reiki practitioner, Pranic healers, and one uncategorised spiritual healer. Yet all of these interventions gave me relief. Together with attention to stress management in the form of holidays, work reduction, and meditation, the frequency and severity of these attacks have greatly diminished over the last two decades.

What interested me was that each of these treatment modalities has its own rationale for working. Scientific evidence for the effectiveness of some of these treatments is at best scant and in some therapies, non-existent. Yet in my case, all of them were effective. The respective practitioners were running successful businesses based on their techniques. Presumably, other people were also finding their treatments helpful.

While the scientific explanation for each modality differed, the art of healing seemed much the same for all of these diverse practitioners. Each practitioner showed a caring attitude and confidence in a successful outcome.

I believe that hope, faith, and love are the foundations of healing. Medicine has long been considered both an art and a science, but in this age of rapid growth in science and technology, the art of medicine has received less emphasis.

While the science of medicine addresses disease, the art of medicine addresses the patient. A great heart surgeon can perform not only a technically good bypass operation but can also show genuine interest in the patient and his or her family, reassure them all, and keep them informed of the patient's progress.

The art of medicine is often summarised by the words 'bedside manner. In 1988, Dr. Herbert Benson founded the Mind/Body Medical Institute at Harvard in order to study the power of belief and therapeutic relationship on health outcomes and started the process

DR. PETER L. JOHNSTON

of putting it on a scientific footing.[1] Its essence, as I see it, remains unchanged from two thousand years ago when Paul of Tarsus wrote, *"Meanwhile these three remain: faith, hope and love. And the greatest of these is love."*[2]

Hope

The value of hope can be seen more clearly by contrasting it with its opposite—hopelessness. People who view their conditions as hopeless believe they are certain losers. They carry a belief that they cannot win. Such belief, attracting the accompanying emotions of fear, depression, and despair, ensures failure by bringing to fruition the very result expected.

It is vital in any healing process for hope to be rekindled. In medical practice it is easy to give people hope and confidence about overcoming diseases and problems for which there is a ready remedy. It is more challenging to offer hope to people with chronic illness where there are no cures. It is even harder when the problem is metastatic cancer, a problem that carries the additional burden of negative cultural beliefs. In the Australian native culture, the ultimate tribal punishment was 'pointing the bone.' It involved banishment from the tribe and usually death. When I was an intern in the 1960s, a young Aboriginal youth was admitted to our public hospital with an anxiety state. The *kadaicha* man had pointed the bone at him. The young man believed he had only six weeks to live. At the time, it made no sense to me. Along with other colleagues, we thought it was a silly delusion which psychotherapy would remove. Unfortunately, despite medical and psychiatric ministrations, the young man died six weeks later. Post-mortem examination provided no clear cause for his death. It was a memorable example of both the power of belief and the absence of hope.

Once cancer has reached the stage of being 'inoperable,' it tends to be seen as 'incurable.' As a result, people with metastatic cancer have the task of not only overcoming their own fears and doubts, but also overcoming their society's attitude of hopelessness. Sometimes their physicians and oncologists share the same pessimism.

The Institute of Noetic Sciences collected more than 3,500 accounts of spontaneous remission from 830 medical journals in more than twenty languages. The first records started in 1846 and the last in the early 1990s. *Spontaneous remission* is a term used by the medical profession to describe a remission or cure that cannot be accounted for by current medical treatment. Remissions were reported to occur in almost every disease, including every form of cancer.[3]

Stages of hope

Once hope enters the picture, possibilities emerge. Cancer patients often show early signs of hope by displaying a fighting attitude. They want to 'beat it.' Fighters generally live longer than those who succumb to feelings of hopelessness and helplessness. While they live longer, they rarely attain a full remission. Part of the reason for this is that their hope is conflicting with their belief. Their hope is not to die, but their belief system has not changed from the cultural one that expects death. Because it is driven by fear, this level of hope is fragile and can be easily undermined by a setback, a recurrence, or a negative statement from a doctor.

Nevertheless, it is a positive start, and from this, higher forms of hope can emerge—forms of hope that are driven by love rather than fear. Love's way focuses not on the disease but on more positive hopes:

- hope for a better quality of life
- hope for a better understanding of life
- hope for a better understanding of one's self
- hope for attaining a state of self-love and self-acceptance
- hope for healing and transformation

The journey of healing and transformation requires a considerable degree of courage as it involves an honest assessment of one's life, with its successes, disappointments and personal animosities. It entails a commitment to address all the unfinished issues of one's life, emotional, physical and spiritual.

DR. PETER L. JOHNSTON

The foundation for hope is living in the present. The present time is all we really have but our minds like to take us into the past or future, where we cannot act. I used to think meditation was relaxing and chilling out but it is actually about tuning in—not tuning out. It is about giving one's full attention to what is here and now. Over the last few decades the word '*mindfulness*' has been used to describe this attitude. Mindfulness is not about fighting or avoiding death. Rather than looking to escape death, the focus is more on examining life and death in more detail with the goal of understanding more.

People who learn to "take each day one at a time," maximising the happiness they can bring to the day, not only improve their quality of life but sometimes increase the quantity of it too. By keeping their mind on the present, they leave less space for the thoughts of hopelessness about the future. Pessimistic ruminations about the future not only feed the illness but also sabotage the potential happiness of the remaining days of so many people. Some are even grateful for the cancer that pushed them into this new state of being. I have known dying patients express their gratitude for the learning that cancer brought them. These people may have died, but the inspiration they gave to those around them will never be lost.

One survivor who remains an inspiration to many is Ian Gawler. Ian was a veterinary surgeon and athlete who developed bone cancer in his twenties. His leg was removed at the groin in an attempt to save his life. The cancer soon recurred in his lungs, where X-rays showed bony growths. At one stage, he was coughing up bone chips in his phlegm. He was told his chances of survival were one in a thousand. In the 1970s, Dr. Ainslie Meares pioneered the use of meditation in the treatment of cancer, and Ian became one of his clients. Ian's journey led him thereafter to various healers, psychic surgeons, dietary regimes, and a meeting with an Indian avatar who told him he was healed. From there on, he improved and has been in complete remission for over thirty years.

Soon after he went into remission, Ian started a centre for cancer patients. Over a period of nearly thirty years, thousands of people have been through his centre, learning to meditate, eat more wholesomely, and change their thinking. I have heard him speak of "five levels of hope," and his vast experience in this area has been a help to me in understanding my own patients and their struggles with hope.[4]

Faith

Faith is the substance of things hoped for,
the evidence of things not seen.[5]

If hope opens the door to healing, faith gives more certainty to this hope. Faith is a stronger expression. Faith is a belief that the things we hope for, especially healing of our diseases, are on the way, that the result is a foregone conclusion. As we say in Australia, "She'll be right, mate. No worries."

Using the cancer example, patients' hopes of survival can turn to faith, which can grow in strength as the following realisations occur in their lives:

- They develop an understanding that incur-ability does not mean unheal-ability. The body can heal where doctors cannot cure.
- Cancer cells are immature and only live a few weeks. It is not necessary to eliminate them all. Changing their pattern of formation is what will heal.
- Cancer may be sending a message that there is something amiss.
- If so, the reason for the cancer is known within and can be accessed.
- Inner knowing of that reason can lead to changing one's life to act in accordance with this knowledge. This can render the message obsolete.
- Such inner transformation can change the pattern producing the cancer cells. New cancer cells cease production. The old cancer cells continue to live only their short life span. So the cancer goes into remission.

Realisations lead to experiences, which in turn lead to greater faith. Positive change can occur when patients with cancer experience the following:

- Meet or read about people who have survived metastatic cancer.
- Feel a calming of the inner panic and fear.
- Notice a change in their attitudes and outlook.
- Start to see positive changes in their lives and start to change the downward spiral of illness into a movement toward health.
- Notice any physical improvement.

All such experiences strengthen faith and can lead to an expectation that healing is on the way. While I have seen individual examples of this, scientifically, the jury is still out on the power of faith to modify cancer. Nevertheless, prolonged depression was shown to double the risk of cancer developing, suggesting that a positive outlook lessens the risk of getting cancer in the first place.[6]

In the therapeutic setting, there are five areas where faith is helpful, if not essential, for a successful outcome in treating any illness.

1. Client's faith in the practitioner

It is important that the client is at least open to the possibility that healing might result from a consultation with a therapist. The man who sits in my consulting room and tells me his wife made the appointment for him and drove him to see me does not fill me with great optimism. Sometimes positives come from such consultations because at least his wife has faith in the work I do. Obviously, it would be preferable to have somebody who has actively chosen to seek help and who is prepared to make changes if necessary. This is why personal recommendation is the best form of marketing. The client who has profited as a result of a therapist's help will be a good advocate for the practitioner. And it comes with no advertising costs.

THE EAGLE'S WAY

Clients who arrive with positive expectations have already started to exercise faith. They have come believing that healing is possible. As long as nothing is said or done to dash this optimism, the client will probably do well—even though the remedy given by the practitioner might be "only a placebo" in the eyes of a mainstream physician.

The word *placebo* is a Latin word meaning 'I shall please.' It was first used to describe the use of harmless remedies given to hypochondriacs to make them feel cared for and to satisfy their need for recognition and treatment. It still has negative connotations in conventional medicine because the word implies that it has no scientific validity. A placebo is only effective because a person believes in it.

Placebos find their main function in double-blind trials. What has proved interesting is that double-blind clinical trials have reported placebos producing improvement in up to 75 per cent of patients. In most trials, the figure varies between 25 and 75 per cent. Others have put it between zero and 100 percent.[7] So at times a new medication may have to perform very well to achieve better results than the placebo.

Placebo is not limited to medications either. In 2002, a randomized controlled trial was conducted on 180 patients with osteoarthritis of the knee. One group received arthroscopic debridement, another arthroscopic lavage and a third group had placebo surgery in the form of skin incisions but no arthroscopy. At no point did either of the intervention groups report less pain or better function than the placebo group. It was a very disappointing result for the surgical team who concluded that arthroscopy was not of value in osteoarthritis of the knee. Yet it was not so disappointing for some of the recipients of placebo surgery, who were able to walk and move in ways they could not do prior to their placebo surgery.[8]

2. Client's faith in the practitioner's healing method

In my experience, people respond better to herbs if they have come from countries where herbs have a long history of use. Similarly, my

DR. PETER L. JOHNSTON

patients have tended to get better results with homeopathic remedies if they themselves or their forebears have used homeopathics in the past.

I first started giving out Bach flower essences to patients about thirty years ago after I heard a veterinary surgeon praise them. He had found them a great help for pets with their emotional problems. In my enthusiasm for using something safe, I gave them to people of all ages. However, over time, I realised they worked wonderfully for babies with colic, feeding, and sleeping problems. They worked well for behavioural problems in young children. They were effective for sensitive adults and those on the path of self-development. But they did little for my other patients, some of whom thought there was too little in them to do any good. The essences possibly worked well in the former groups because these patients lacked the scepticism that blocks faith.

Many of my patients who presented with colds or flu expected me to prescribe antibiotics. Their faith was in antibiotics and they got worse when they did not receive them. Antibiotics are for bacterial infections, not viral ones, but my intellectual understanding was not the important factor. The belief of the person with the illness is more important. If a person believes their cold will get worse without antibiotics, it seems to do that.

Stewart Wolf, an American psychologist and pioneer in mind-body medicine, did interesting work on the effect of drugs on the stomach by using measurements of the internal muscular wave patterns there. He found that his patient's expectations overrode the effects of drugs. Ipecac is given to patients to induce vomiting, while atropine is given to reduce secretions and reduce the risk of vomiting. When he administered ipecac to a patient but told him it was atropine, the patient's stomach showed none of the expected ipecac effects.[9]

Patient expectations of treatment can also have a negative impact—referred to as a *nocebo* effect. A randomised controlled clinical trial to test the efficacy of two chemotherapy protocols for stomach cancer was conducted at several British hospitals in the days before it was considered unethical to use placebo in cancer. Four hundred and eleven patients with stomach cancer were divided into three groups. Two groups received active chemotherapy while the control group received injections of normal saline solution every three weeks. In the control group receiving the placebo injections of saline, the following occurred:

- 34.6 per cent experienced nausea related to their injections.
- 21.5 per cent reported treatment-related vomiting.
- 30.8 per cent reported hair loss.

It would appear the patients' belief that they were receiving chemotherapy was sufficient for them to experience the common side effects of the treatment.[10]

In our Western culture, our faith and trust is placed in conventional scientific medicine. As a doctor, my first treatment option is usually drugs or surgery, which is what most people expect when they go to a doctor.

Nevertheless, the pattern is changing. There is a growing interest in vitamins, herbs, and minerals and a respect for alternative approaches to health care. However, there will still be a need and respect for the old ways too. Where possible, I use methods and supplements in accord with the patient's own belief system.

Notwithstanding what I have written about the deficiencies of conventional medicine in the previous chapters, its benefits far outstrip its limitations. I have great respect for mainstream medicine and what it offers. I also respect its need to remain scientifically based. Otherwise, it runs the risk of regressing to the unscientific standards of nineteenth-century therapeutics. So unless CAM therapies can find scientific verification, they will remain under the category of complementary therapies.

I have had an interest in CAM therapies for thirty years and have been comfortable using them alongside mainstream therapies. Despite my passion for complementary medicine, I have never been tempted to specialise in them. I have remained a general practitioner, utilising virtually all aspects of conventional treatment.

3. Practitioners' faith in their own methods

A practitioner's trust in his or her own healing method is essential and plays a vital role in the placebo response. The effect of a doctor giving a pill to a patient is in itself an act carrying a certain amount of power and capacity to heal. As mentioned previously, this placebo response can result in improvement in the patient's condition.

When I first started as a locum in general practice in the mid-sixties, Dr. Jim recommended that I continue his custom of giving calcium injections to his Mediterranean patients. He justified his treatment with the words, "They believe in injections rather than pills." His patients seemed happy with these injections from me while I worked there. Yet when I did the same thing in my own practice, they did not work. I suspect the difference between the two practices was that Dr. J believed in his calcium injections whereas I did not.

Dr. Larry Dossey, in his book *Healing Words,* quoted studies suggesting that physicians' beliefs could affect the results of double-blind trials even though neither the physician nor the patients knew whether they were receiving the active ingredient or the placebo.[11] In three double-blind studies testing the efficacy of vitamin E in angina pectoris, one doctor who was enthusiastic about vitamin E found it significantly more effective than the placebo.[12] At the same time, two studies conducted by sceptics showed no effect.[13] A similar result occurred when meprobamate was given a double-blind trial by two physicians. Meprobamate was found to be significantly more powerful than placebo, but only for the doctor who believed in it. The more detached doctor's trial showed no effect at all.[14]

The practitioners' faith and trust in their techniques, modalities, or remedies are crucial. Whether they use drugs, surgery, acupuncture needles, chants, tom-toms, or chicken gizzards may be less important than the trust they have in them. The practitioner's faith provides an energy that is picked up by the client, more often subconsciously than consciously, and this enhances the client's own faith.

THE EAGLE'S WAY

4. Practitioner's faith in their client's capacity for self-healing

It is sometimes overlooked that clients actually heal themselves regardless of which healing modality is used. All healing is self-healing. When doctors suture a wound, they bring the edges of the wound together, but it is the body that actually knits the edges into unified, functional tissue. When orthopaedic surgeons apply plaster casts for fractures, they are bringing bone fragments together so the body can heal itself more effectively. Even when they insert synthetic hips or knees, they are relying on the body's healing response to incorporate those prostheses. Any drugs, herbs, or vitamins are really only aids to the body's own healing capacity.

All cells go through the life cycle of birth, life, and death. The life cycle of skin cells is only about six weeks—less if sunburnt. Until recently, nerve cells were believed to be the exception. Once damaged, as in spinal injury or stroke, the nerve cells do not seem to regenerate. In the late nineties, a team at Salk Laboratories in California found a way to stain brain cells in such a way the marker only gets taken up at the moment the cell comes into being, when it lights up the microscope. Using this technique, they were able to demonstrate new brain cells coming into existence even in people who were dying.[15]

In his remarkable bestseller titled *The Brain That Changes Itself,* Dr. Norman Doidge told the story of Pedro Bach-y-Rita, a widowed poet and scholar who in 1959, at the age of sixty-five, had a severe stroke that left him paralysed down one side and unable to speak. Rather than leave him in a nursing home, his eldest son, George, a medical student, brought him home to Mexico. With the help of the gardener, George was able to lift him for showering and toileting. George bought him knee pads and encouraged him to crawl, leaning his weak side against the wall. He also devised games to strengthen Pedro's weak arm and hand, and Pedro was conscientious with the exercises.

Wanting to resume writing, Pedro would hold his middle finger over the desired key and then drop his arm on it. After hours of practice, he could drop just his wrist over the key and eventually his fingers one at a time until he could type again. At the end of twelve months, he could stand and walk and returned to teaching full-time.

He remarried, travelled, and hiked until his death from a heart attack at seventy-two.[16] A post-mortem examination still showed catastrophic damage to his brain stem. Yet somehow with the work Pedro had done, his brain had reorganized itself to re-establish function.[17]

Pedro's younger son, Paul, has become one of the great pioneers in a new arena of medical science called neuroplasticity, which is the study of the way in which the brain and nervous system changes structure with different activities so as to be better suited to the task and how other parts can take over when certain parts of the brain are damaged.[18]

Medical textbooks tend to avoid the words 'uniformly fatal' in describing an incurable, lethal disease because there always seems to be the odd person who breaks the rules and gets better even where the general prognosis is extremely gloomy.

A much more positive rule to be guided by is this: "Nothing is impossible." The human body, which created itself in all its complexity from one single cell, seems to be capable of healing any disease if it is given the appropriate conditions.[3] Among the appropriate conditions required are adequate nutrients, both physical and mental—and the latter includes a sense of faith and trust in the capacity of the human organism to heal itself.

5. Faith in the capacity of the practitioner-client relationship to effect healing

The interaction between the client and the therapist can itself catalyse healing. People researching the placebo response have found that patients who are encouraged to explain their discomfort to doctors fare better than those who are just given a prescription.[19]

Characteristics enhancing the placebo response were the following:

- Sincere accurate empathy from the doctor
- Warmth and genuineness on the doctor's part
- trust in the doctor by the patient[20]

THE EAGLE'S WAY

Long consultations resulted in better outcomes, less medications, and more patient and doctor satisfaction, according to a survey done in 2002.[21]

When both parties are relaxed and share a good rapport, spontaneous words and conversations often emerge. These can trigger insights that can lead to changes and healing. Healing is by no means a one-way street either. At times, a throwaway line or a chance comment from a patient has had a significant impact on the way I have dealt with a problem in my own life. At other times, my words have spontaneously flowed on an issue involving the client. When the client has left, the impact of what I have said suddenly hits me. I have realised the message is every bit as important for me as it was for the client. It is a timely reminder to practise what I preach, confirming the truth behind the saying that "we teach best what we most need to learn."

The critical point in healing comes when a patient's belief in disease changes to a belief in health. This fundamental step, where the patient starts to believe that he or she is going to get better, starts an energy chain that leads to more positive emotions. These emotions in turn lead to an alteration in the body chemicals and ultimately in the cellular structure.

Love

Love is indeed the most important of the three components of healing. It is difficult for clients to have faith in practitioners who show no love or passion for their work or for their clients. Rapport is an important ingredient in the establishment of faith, as shown in the surveys.[19,20,21]

The word "love" can lead to confusion because of the many meanings attached to it. In the clinical setting, it does not mean hugging every client—although it may be okay to do so if it feels appropriate for both client and therapist. It certainly does not mean making love with patients. Sex with clients brings a load of other complications into the relationship, one of which can be the loss of one's licence to practise.

DR. PETER L. JOHNSTON

Nor does love mean pleasing clients. Much of the time it will be doing so but frequently caring brings discomfort. Short-term pain for long-term gain is a maxim in health care. Painful or uncomfortable procedures are often the least painful way to go in the long term. Lancing boils to allow toxins to escape is a process that can apply just as appropriately to emotional and mental toxins as it does to physical ones. Saying no to patients who want something contravening a practitioner's integrity may sometimes be necessary. The 'tough love' required in helping drug addicts may appear at times unloving. Yet love can be expressed in many ways: withholding as well as giving, constructive criticism as well as praise, and maintaining discipline as well as having fun.

A working definition of love in health care

Love is too vast a concept to be captured in a definition, but in the context of a consultation with a health-care practitioner, the word 'compassion' comes closest. Carl Rogers, a pioneer of humanistic psychology, used the term "unconditional positive regard" to describe the appropriate attitude. The importance of regarding both the patient and the problem in a positive light cannot be understated. The extent to which this sense of caring and appreciation for the client can be maintained is an indicator of the degree of help the therapist is giving. *Unconditional* means therapists maintain a sense of care and appreciation for their clients. At no time do they judge their clients.

Using empathy, therapists 'feel with' their clients and try to understand the presenting problem from the client's perspective. When I do this, I frequently find I would probably have taken the same course of action they did. "Walking in another's moccasins" is a way of developing compassion and unconditional acceptance of another.

Positive is sometimes a difficult state to achieve as it requires an optimistic outlook toward both the patient and the patient's presenting problems. Many doctors have clients they describe as 'heart-sink patients.' I only have to see certain names on my appointment list to have a sinking feeling. I expect they are going to come with a load

THE EAGLE'S WAY

of problems and take them back home again. They will be deaf to any advice I give in the course of our consultation. I know they can be healed, but I question whether that is what they actually desire. Is their illness still serving an important purpose in their lives? Is it gaining them attention they still need? Are they ready to let it go? These people challenge my capacity to maintain unconditional positive regard—as do angry, critical, or unappreciative clients.

Regard is about giving attention and respect to one's client. It really implies the client has the undivided attention of the therapist for the time he or she is in the consulting room. However, even with the best of intentions, some distracting thoughts can enter: "I hope I'm doing this properly. He reminds me of Fred, the class clown of primary school. I hope she doesn't go on and on about this problem." Provided that such thoughts are only transitory, I can still create a welcome space. The expression 'quality time' expresses this concept of total, undivided attention. This form of attention is empowering to the person receiving it.

Quality time, which is unconditionally caring in nature, connects, lifts, and heals. Providing it in a therapeutic space creates a receptacle wherein clients can feel safe to express their truths. When they can share their painful secrets and have them acknowledged without judgement, it frees them to accept themselves as they are. This in turn allows them to love themselves more. This self-love reconnects them to themselves and renders them more whole, more healed.

Scientific studies

As noted earlier, healing and wholeness were derived from the same word.[22] Healing is about wholeness. The force bringing about wholeness is love. Love unites people—whether it is romantic love, love for friends or family, love for a cause or organisation, or love for a sport or hobby. Love brings people together and creates bonds. Love for one's self creates inner peace.

Research is showing a connection between disease and the lack of love in a person's life.[22] Studies have shown isolation to be associated with a higher incidence of heart disease,[23,24,25] peptic ulcers,[26]

DR. PETER L. JOHNSTON

and tuberculosis.[27] The rate of complications in pregnancy is higher in those who do not have a supporting partner,[28,29] while people who are HIV positive show a higher rate of conversion to clinical AIDS in the absence of support.[30]

Other studies have shown a lower rate of serious illness in those who have had satisfactory relationships with their parents,[31,32] while those who have a good relationship with their spouses show a lower incidence of illness generally.[33,34,35] Supportive relationships within the community have been shown to be health protective,[36,37] and other studies have shown the health benefits of having a pet around the home.[38,39] The value of group support for patients with melanoma[40] and breast cancer[41] has been demonstrated in clinical trials.

Dr. Dean Ornish conducted the first trial that proved lifestyle changes were capable of reversing heart disease. His initial trial followed forty-eight patients with significant coronary artery disease. Their level of pathology was confirmed by coronary angiography—both before and after the trial. The control group had no lifestyle intervention whereas the treatment group had a low-fat vegetarian diet, exercise, yoga, meditation, and group support. After one year, there was a 91 per cent reduction in the frequency of anginal pain in the intervention group, compared with an increase of 165 per cent in the control group. Angiography showed an 82 per cent improvement in the intervention group as against 53 per cent deterioration in the control group. After three years, the difference between the two groups was even greater.[42,43]

While the medical profession directed their focus to diet and lifestyle as the significant factors in producing these outstanding results, Dean Ornish himself had his own ideas. In his book *Love and Survival*, he wrote the following:

> *I have no intention of diminishing the power of diet and exercise or, for that matter, drugs and surgery. There is more evidence now than ever before demonstrating how simple changes in diet and lifestyle can cause significant improvements in health and wellbeing.*[44]

As important as these are, I have found that perhaps the most powerful intervention—and the most meaningful for me—and for most of the people with whom I work, including staff and patients—is the HEALING POWER OF LOVE and INTIMACY, and the emotional and spiritual transformation that often result from these.[45]

And it made such a difference that many insurance companies are paying for their clients to attend his courses. As Dean Ornish put it, "*They are finding it is good business to help patients open their hearts.*"[46]

Visually impressive is the work of Dr. Masaru Emoto, a Japanese researcher. He froze various samples of water and photographed the crystals. Untreated distilled water showed a vague circular structure. When hostile words were addressed to the water prior to freezing, the crystalline structure was reminiscent of a section of a hot mud pool. On the other hand, when words of love and appreciation were given to the water, the resultant crystals showed a beautiful hexagonal crystalline structure like a glistening diamond brooch.

Dr. Emoto's photographs suggest that water is alive and responsive to human thoughts and emotions. Because water makes up 70 to 80 per cent of the human body, it seems reasonable to assume our bodies respond in similar fashion to love.[47]

The importance of self-love in health

The word *holy* used to mean *being whole*, but nowadays it carries an air of being sanctimonious. The expression "having one's act together" gives a better idea of wholeness. It describes people who have competence, confidence, and a sense of direction. People who have purpose in their lives could be described as having self-esteem without arrogance.

At its highest level, self-esteem could be described as a state of unconditional love for one's self. This means loving ourselves just the way we are, not because we have fulfilled criteria set by our families or workplaces. This state of unconditional self-love is fed from within. If we could give ourselves the same acceptance, forgiveness, and unconditional love that we so often bestow on our children and pets, we would be very joyous and happy people. On second thought, if we could give ourselves the unconditional love our dogs bestow on us, we would be even happier.

Self-love would also make us healthier people. I suspect dis-ease would evaporate if we were totally at-ease with ourselves. If we loved ourselves unconditionally, we would not have to spend so much time harshly criticising ourselves over what we 'should have done' when we probably never wanted to do many of those things in the first place.

By accepting our clients with unconditional love, we help them to see it in themselves. Louise Hay, a popular writer on the subject of metaphysics, wrote a paragraph that I have found very helpful in approaching patients: *"No matter where you are in life, no matter what you've contributed to creating, no matter what's happening, you are always doing the best you can with the understanding, awareness and knowledge that you have at the time."*[48]

In reality, there are no mistakes—there is only learning. Children learn to walk by tumbling and falling, and they do not castigate themselves for doing so. As a result, they learn quickly. Learning to cook a medium-rare steak on the barbecue usually involves charring it and undercooking it until there is enough experience to get the timing right.

Anecdote

It was thirty-seven years ago when I first discovered the power of love in healing. Our first son was born prematurely after a difficult pregnancy and an even more traumatic labour for my wife. It was expected that our son would not survive, so my wife and I were advised by the paediatrician and staff not to see him in case we became too attached to him. It was considered the kindest course for everybody involved. Our son only lived three days. Neither my wife nor I really accepted his death. At times, I still feel grief over his death.

THE EAGLE'S WAY

Fortunately, another opportunity presented itself four years later. After an even worse pregnancy, much of it spent in hospital, my wife delivered a baby boy who was not only premature but who was less developed than most babies of the same chronological age in utero. This time, we spent much of our time next to our son's incubator. We talked to him and let him know how much we loved him and wanted him to stay. He survived and is now himself a health practitioner.

I was reminded of this when I saw a beautiful photo on the Internet. It came from an article called "The Rescuing Hug." The article details the first week of life for a set of twins. Apparently, both were in their respective incubators. One of them was not expected to live. A nurse ignored the hospital rules and placed the babies in one incubator. When they were placed together, the healthier of the two threw an arm over her sister in an endearing embrace. The smaller baby's heart rate stabilised, and her temperature rose to normal. The twins and now twenty-four and healthy.

CHAPTER 6

An Age Of Separation

The ways in which mainstream, alternative, and holistic medicine have evolved are easier to understand when viewed from a historical perspective. While the art of health care has changed little over millennia, the science of health care has undergone dramatic change over five hundred years—particularly over the last two centuries.

A Brief History of Medicine

From earliest recorded history, healthcare went hand in hand with spirituality and tribal religion. Primitive peoples saw disease as being inflicted upon them from the spiritual world by gods or by evil spirits. The shaman, witch doctor, or medicine man treated the ailing member of the tribe by using herbs, chants, talismans, and rituals aimed at pleasing the gods. Even in Greece, the cradle of Western civilisation, people would come to the temple of Aesculepius, the god of healing. There, they would sleep and allow their dreams to point the way to health. Health care in Europe in the Middle Ages centred around the monasteries, where nuns and monks attended the sick and dying.

In contrast to this tradition, the major advances in Western medicine have come with the separation of health care from the world of spirits and religion. Separation and togetherness are, of course, relative terms. Even now in the twenty-first century, there are many hospitals and hospices run by religious orders. Similarly, there are physicians who incorporate religion into their work. Nevertheless, in comparison with earlier times, separation of health care and religion has been a distinctive feature of modern Western medicine.

Origins of Western medicine

Hippocrates, a Greek physician in the fifth century BC, is honoured as the first person in the Western world to question the spiritual origin of disease. He postulated disease to be caused by earthly influences. He wrote, "*Every disease has its own nature and arises from external causes.*"[1] He paid particular attention to a patient's diet, occupation, and the climate of his or her life, both geographic and astrological. His theoretical conception was known as the *humoral* theory. He believed health to require equilibrium between four bodily fluids— blood, phlegm, black bile, and yellow bile. Although he excluded the gods from his list of disease producers, he acknowledged the importance of ethics in health care. His Hippocratic oath is still administered to new graduates in medicine.

The period of stagnation

A clear and accurate understanding of human anatomy was essential for health care to have a scientific basis, and this could only be gained by dissecting human bodies. Although ancient Egyptians preserved separate organs as well as complete bodies, there is no evidence they studied human remains in order to better understand human anatomy or disease. The ancient Greeks and Indians both cremated their dead without autopsies, while the Romans, Chinese, and Muslims all had taboos about opening dead bodies. The Mediaeval Christian Church also forbade autopsies.

As a result, medical science in the fifteenth century was based on the textbooks of Galen, a Greek physician of the second century AD. Galen had based his medical system on the teachings of Hippocrates, combined with an understanding of philosophy based on Plato and Aristotle. Galen saw anatomy as fundamental to medical knowledge. However, he was physician to the Roman emperor of the time, Marcus Aurelius, and his later successors, who did not permit human dissection. Consequently, Galen's knowledge of anatomy was drawn from his own dissection of animals.

With the fall of Rome, scholarship seemed to lose its status. Experiment and originality were discouraged, if not actually punished. Tradition ruled. The Christian concept of disease went back to the spiritual world. Sickness was a punishment for sin. Treatment dictated repentance, prayer, and penance. Nevertheless, as well as caring for the sick, the church transcribed and preserved the ancient Greek manuscripts on healing, suggesting they had not entirely discarded the concept of more earthly causes for disease.

Progress at last

The Renaissance brought not only the rebirth of Greek and Roman culture but a total change in outlook. There arose an interest in escaping the limits of tradition and the restrictions of religious dogma and doctrines. There was an enthusiasm to explore new fields.

One such field was anatomy. Leonardo da Vinci did a number of anatomical drawings based on his own dissections, which caused some difficulties between Rome and his patrons, the Medici family. Living a little farther away from Rome was Andreas Vesalius (1514-64), who is considered the 'father of anatomy.' His work, translated as *The Seven Books on the Structure of the Human Body*, was printed in 1543.[2] In it, he showed conclusively that Galen's anatomy belonged to the realms of veterinary rather than medical science. His close attention to detail laid the foundations for a science of medicine based on careful observation.

While normal anatomy was established quickly, it took many autopsies before there was an adequate understanding of human disease. The "father of pathology" was Giovanni Morgagni. In 1761, he wrote *On the Seats and Causes of Diseases as Investigated by Anatomy*. In this work, he documented the symptoms and physical findings in seven hundred patients and then compared them with what he found in the same patients at autopsy.

A great pioneer in physiology was William Harvey (1578-1657), who used a series of experiments and careful measurement to establish the one-way nature of the circulation of blood. Galen had taught of the ebb and flow of blood like the tides. Harvey realised the heart valves would force blood to flow one way only. Although he could not prove the connection between arteries and veins, his theory was proven soon after his death when Malpighi, using early microscopes, demonstrated the existence of the tiny capillaries in the lungs and tissues.

The discovery of microorganisms

The invention of the microscope brought new discoveries, not only in anatomy but also more importantly in pathology. As early as the mid-1670s, a Dutch microscope-maker described bacteria and protozoa and presented his findings to the Royal Society. However, nearly two hundred years were to elapse before the significance of his observations were to be recognised.

Varro, a Roman writer, mentioned the possibility of disease being caused by invisible particles as early as the first century BC. No doubt the prevalence of plagues in Europe stimulated similar ideas in the centuries before microscopes. However, not until the mid-nineteenth century did conclusive evidence come into being.

In 1848, Ignaz Semmelweiss, an obstetrician, reduced the maternal mortality in his ward from 18.27 to 1.27 per cent by insisting all medical students washed their hands in chlorinated lime before they examined expectant mothers. Between 1865 and 1869, Joseph Lister reduced the mortality after surgical amputations from 45 to 15 per cent by introducing carbolic acid as an antiseptic in surgery.

These major breakthroughs in the war against inflammation were underpinned by the work of Louis Pasteur (1822-95). Pasteur, a French chemist, pioneered the concept of taking scientific experimentation out of the laboratory into the field. In so doing, he proved bacteria to be the agents causing putrefaction and fermentation as well as human and animal diseases.

DR. PETER L. JOHNSTON

Joseph Lister was aware of Pasteur's work. Unlike Semmelweiss, he knew what he was fighting. By the end of the century, the use of antiseptic as a front-line agent in surgery gave way to asepsis, the technique whereby microorganisms are excluded by sterilising all instruments and gowns worn by operating theatre personnel. The conquest of infection together with the discovery of ether as a safe anaesthetic in the mid-nineteenth century transformed surgery. With the capacity to combat blood loss with transfusion in the twentieth century, surgery became the relatively safe procedure we now know.

The discovery of microbes as causes of disease was given further impetus by the German physician Robert Koch (1843-1910), who created a procedure for determining which microorganisms caused each specific disease. By the end of the nineteenth century, the causes of most infectious diseases had been classified. With the discovery of sulphonamides and penicillin in the twentieth century, bacterial diseases could be successfully treated.[3]

The state of medicine in 1965

In the mid-1960s, the wisdom of Hippocrates seemed self-evident. Each disease had been shown to have its own nature, and most had been shown to arise from external causes:

- Acute infections arose from microorganisms, mainly bacteria and viruses.
- Chronic infections like tuberculosis and syphilis were caused by bacteria.
- Chronic tropical diseases like malaria and schistosomiasis were due to parasites.
- Chemical trauma was caused by poisoning, addictions, and the side effects of medications.
- Physical traumas arose from (a) direct impact, mainly motor vehicle injuries and sports, (b) excess heat or cold, (c) exposure to radiation or electrocution, (d) exposure to too much pressure in blast injuries, and (e) too rapid decompression after diving.

THE EAGLE'S WAY

- Nutritional diseases arose from (a) too much food of poor quality in the Western world, (b) starvation in the Third World, and (c) vitamin deficiencies.
- Allergic disorders were caused by exposure to certain grasses, foods, pollens, and moulds (and a microbe called the house dust mite).
- Cancer and tumours arose from a number of environmental factors:
  a) Cigarette smoke in cancers of lung, lips, tongue, throat, and larynx
  b) Aniline dyes in bladder cancers
  c) Excessive radiation in leukaemias
  d) Excessive exposure to the sun in skin cancers
  e) Asbestos in mesothelioma (a cancer of the lung)
  f) Viruses found in many warts and some tumours

- Endocrine diseases arose from (a) a Western diet, which was implicated in adult onset diabetes, and (b) iodine deficiency in thyroid disease.
- Congenital diseases arose from viral diseases, in particular rubella, which was found to produce birth defects. The drug thalidomide was also implicated in congenital defects.

While there were still chronic infections, tumours, endocrine disorders, and congenital diseases for which medical science had no known cause and a category called *idiopathic,* which doctors translate as 'cause unknown,' there was an air of optimism about the inevitable outcome. Science would discover the external causes of these conditions, and this would lead to cures.

With external causes so widely accepted as the causes of disease, there was no longer any justification for blaming gods or demons for illness—and certainly no reason to blame the patient. Nevertheless, in their choice of victim, these external causes shared the same randomness as the gods and demons. We still speak of disease as an affliction. The word *affliction* comes from the Latin word *afflictare,* which means 'struck down, harassed, knocked about.'[4] A microbe or a pollutant, like a bus or a murderer, might at any time strike down an innocent victim. This separation of the patient from the cause of his or her illness helped to generate a sense of real compassion for the sick. It also helped stimulate the discovery of many practical aids to easing those afflictions.

Matter as Separate Atoms

A central character in the separation of science from religion, Galileo Galilei (1564-1642) could also lay claim to being the founder of the scientific method. A century before Isaac Newton, he used experiments to check his theoretical deductions on falling objects, motions of projectiles, momentum, and inertia. He built a telescope thirty-two times stronger than any other available in his time. Armed with this, he scoured the heavens and was the first to describe the rings of Saturn, the phases of Venus, and the satellites of Jupiter. He described spots on the Sun and noted the Milky Way to be comprised of many individual stars. He saw the surface of the moon as being irregular, not smooth. His astronomical observations confirmed the Copernican theory of a solar system wherein the planets, including Earth, revolved around the Sun. These latter two discoveries contradicted the literal interpretation of the Bible. As a result, the Inquisition forced Galileo to recant his claims, and he spent the last eight years of his life under house arrest.

Galileo, together with the other great scientists of the seventeenth century, Isaac Newton, Robert Boyle, Christian Huygens, and Robert Hooke, believed that matter was composed of small indivisible entities called atoms. The atomic theory was not new. The Greek philosopher Democritus had written about it in the fifth century BC, and it had become a part of the Epicurean philosophy in the fourth and third centuries BC. With the fall of the Roman Empire, the atomic theory faded along with much of the wisdom and knowledge of the ancient world only to be rediscovered during the rebirth of the Greek and Roman culture in Renaissance Europe.

Early in the nineteenth century, Dalton and Avogadro defined molecules as the "smallest particles of a pure compound that retain their characteristic properties." They redefined atoms as "the fundamental building blocks from which molecules are constructed." It made good sense as a theory. To the naked eye, material things are separate from each other. Under the microscope, living organisms could be seen to comprise separate individual cells in relationship with each other. Why would the basic building blocks of matter not be similar—individual and separate atoms in relationship with each other?

It must have seemed common sense to Europeans in the seventeenth, eighteenth, and even early nineteenth century. Their world was one of separate villages and communities whose relationships with each other were less immediate than today. With only horse and cart to traverse the land and sailing ships to cross water, travel was slow. Postage was the only other form of communication, and this was not very fast either. Atoms were the fundamental unit of all physical structures—just like individual human beings were the fundamental unit of humanity. Atoms were seen as separate from other atoms just as humans were separate from other humans. Atoms could group together to form simple molecules just as humans could group together as families, tribes, and communities. Just as individuals could break away from their families and communities without losing their individuality, atoms could remain separate and individual building blocks for the material world.

Separation from the Cosmos

Some refer to astrology as the oldest science on earth. To others, it is a pseudoscience, failing to measure up to the intellectual rigours required of a science. Regardless of its status, astrology had a powerful presence in the ancient world as it connected people to the cosmos. The destinies of individuals and nations could be predicted according to their relationship to the sun, moon, planets, and galaxy. No self-respecting general would go into battle without trying to get an astrological chart on his opponent. The word *universe* is derived from the Latin *universum,* meaning 'whole' or 'combined into one.' The word *cosmos* comes from the Greek word meaning 'order,' the opposite of chaos.[5] Behind astrology was an understanding of an orderly universe in which each individual was a participant. It was a science that connected people to the order existing in the cosmos. Hippocrates was quoted as saying that all physicians should understand astrology with its ramifications for individual health.[6]

Astrology, in the form it was practised in Europe, placed Earth at the centre of the universe. The positions of the Sun, planets, and signs of the zodiac are viewed from the position of a static earth around which the heavens appear to rotate. Galileo's confirmation of the Copernican solar system rendered astrology unscientific. With the development of more powerful telescopes, new planets were discovered in our solar system, rendering astrology even less scientific. With the rise of science, astrology went into decline.

In its place arose the science of astronomy. Astronomy, although being more scientifically accurate than astrology, actually created a greater sense of separation. In place of the science that connected people to the cosmos, astronomy highlighted the vast distances between the earth and other celestial bodies. The distances were too mind-boggling for simple mathematics to handle, so a new measurement called the *light year* was introduced. Because light travels at 186,000 miles per second, the distance travelled in a year is quite significant. Some of our visible stars are hundreds of light years away.

Religious Separation

More prevalent than astrology in giving humanity a sense of place in the cosmos, religion had provided the traditional source of meaning for Europeans. Christianity, with its message of a loving God, had spread rapidly through Europe in the first century AD and had been the dominant religion since the declining years of the Roman Empire. However, by the seventeenth century, church teachings, which reflected a god of fear rather than one of love, had seriously undermined the original message of hope. The fear of burning in hell indefinitely—or in purgatory temporarily—was a potent fear stimulated largely by church's interpretations of scripture.

In the sixteenth century, Pope Leo the tenth built up his church coffers by selling indulgences to the faithful. His promise was that by

THE EAGLE'S WAY

spending money, people could gain plenary indulgences and thereby avoid the fires of hell or purgatory. Such indulgences provoked the fire in Martin Luther, who set out to reform the church but succeeded only in splitting it. With the reformation, the one church divided into many denominations, each claiming to have the truth. Even with their differences, all of them still maintained a sense of separation from the entity referred to as God. Although the scriptures spoke of an imminent or indwelling God, most Christian splinter groups still kept their focus on a transcendent God dwelling in a heaven elsewhere. Not only were the faithful separated from God, they were separated from each other.

Separation of Mind and Body

In the early seventeenth century, Jesuit priests instructed Rene Descartes in the philosophies of Aristotle and Thomas Aquinas. He found neither of them satisfying. Lacking a sense of meaning, he spent the rest of his life formulating a coherent philosophy of life. He discarded any knowledge he could not prove with certainty. This included the evidence from his senses. He even discarded the existence of his own body. He could not be certain his body was not a sensory illusion. However, even uncertainty and doubt involved thinking, so he felt certain about his existence as a thinker. Hence, his famous quote: *Cogito ergo sum,* meaning *"I think, therefore I am."* Because the existence of the mind was self-evident while the body's reality was uncertain, Descartes felt the mind and the body to be radically distinct. He saw the universe as consisting of two different substances: 'mind' or 'thinking substance' and 'matter' or 'physical substance.' He believed physical substances were subject to scientific laws and mathematical formulae. He saw animals, vegetables, and minerals as belonging to this category. For him, humans were the only beings having both substances.

His works were controversial at the time—and remain so. Nevertheless, his efforts to bring together the fields of physics, chemistry, and physiology in a logical way, free of any spiritual explanations, provided a basis for the ensuing scientific approach. The separation of religion and science called for a secular philosophy. Descartes was the first to come forward to fill this vacuum. He is also given much of the credit for the belief in the separation of mind and body. The medical profession in the Western world still keeps psychiatry separate from physical medicine and still uses a secular philosophy as its guiding principle.

Separation from Emotion

Scientific method put its accent on careful, objective observation and experimentation. Inherent to this search for truth was a need to detach from any traditional beliefs, prejudices, passions, and emotional attachments to any specific outcome. The search for truth valued dispassionate, logical thinking and creative thought. Other than a passion for doing the job well, other passions and emotions were considered detrimental to the task.

It is hard to assess the effect of this intellectual approach to medicine because there are other cogent reasons for a physician's detached attitude to patients. Suffering is an inherently emotional event for a patient. Compassion for the sufferer is a necessary part of health care. Yet keeping some sort of boundary between the patient and the doctor is also necessary. Oversensitive health-care workers can find themselves drained and overwhelmed if they allow themselves to participate in their clients' emotions. Clients in panic or severe emotional distress are like people sinking in quicksand. What they need are helpers throwing them a line from solid ground and pulling them out. The last thing they need is their therapist in the quicksand with them.

Another hazard Hippocrates warned about was sex with patients. In the early twentieth century, Sigmund Freud introduced the concept of *transference*. Patients in counselling will often project the roles of parents or intimates onto their therapists. It is a natural part of the healing process, but it is vital for patient and therapist that such transferences are not acted upon. Detachment is important until these projections are withdrawn, which does happen after successful therapy.

All are valid reasons for placing emotions in the back seat of health care. Emotions are also seen as untidy, messy, and sometimes embarrassing and difficult for therapists to handle. Angry or weepy patients can be very unsettling for physicians. Dramatic emotional scenes can put therapists under pressure to act hastily and with less clarity than they might otherwise do.

Separation into Specialities

The industrial revolution that began in the mid-eighteenth century introduced the factory system. When people lived mainly in rural settings, they covered the wide range of farming tasks. Industry demanded specific tasks to be done with a high level of precision. Henry Ford's assembly line for his T-model Ford was a prime example of the benefits of dividing workers into specialised tasks. As medical science and technology became more complex in the twentieth century, specialisation became the dominant pattern in this field too. Surgeons and physicians developed their expertise in smaller, specialized areas that allowed more proficiency in diagnostic and surgical skills.

Analysis

The word *analysis* stems from the Greek word *ana lusis*, which broadly means to 'unloosen or take apart.' It describes the process of separating something into its constituent elements. Analysis stands in contrast to *synthesis*, which is derived from the Greek *sun thusis*, meaning to 'place together.' Synthesis is about putting constituents together to form a connected whole.

The history of modern medicine shows an analytical journey. The human body was initially separated from the soul, spirit, and cosmos—and soon after, it was separated from the mind. Its component parts were then examined and classified. Separating out organs and tissues in the laboratory enabled the accumulation of much knowledge about the way the body functions. Microscopy (and later electron microscopy) allowed a visualisation of the body's cellular constituents. These, too, could be separated out, examined, and used for experiments from which much was learned. Scientists speculated about the fundamental nature of matter, and their experiments suggested the existence of separate atoms as the basic building blocks of life.

In the twentieth century, the medical health-care delivery system reflected this separation by forming specialties and subspecialties to examine and treat each organ or system, including the specialty of psychiatry to treat the mind. Now in the twenty-first century, medical science is exploring the world of molecular biology. The DNA molecule on which the genetic blueprint of life is imprinted is now largely mapped.[7] It is hard to imagine we can get to any smaller aspect of analysis than this.

The New Paradigm

The process of separation and specialisation went hand in hand with medical advances so impressive that the twentieth century must be considered the greatest era of all time for medicine.

Yet in the same century, science itself started to question the basic tenets of separation. Questions arose on a number of fronts, which will be explored in more depth in the following two chapters.

1. Psychologists postulated the unity of mind. Maybe minds were not separate. Dr. C. G. Jung introduced the concept of the collective unconscious.

2. Physicists split the atom and found a quantum field, a unified field of energy instead of the expected separate particles of matter.

3. Discoveries in medicine and physics suggested that mind and matter were not separate.

4. Biologists studied ecology and found a deeper interrelationship between all aspects of life than had been hitherto understood.

5. The discovery of the hologram provided a new concept of the whole contained in each of the parts.

CHAPTER 7

The New Paradigm Of Consciousness

A *paradigm shift* is "*a radical change in underlying beliefs or theory.*" It was a term coined by T. S. Kuhn (1922-96), an American philosopher of science.[1] By its very nature, a paradigm is more an unconscious belief, one taken for granted as a feature of reality. There has been a major shift from a belief in separation to an understanding that perhaps beneath the appearances of separation lies unity—in consciousness, mind, and matter.

The Collective Unconscious

Jung's view of the psyche was a holistic one, seeing the individual mind not as a totally separate entity but as part of a 'universal mind.' Jung saw each individual as being plugged into a universal source, taking from it in a mostly unconscious way. He expressed the relationship between the individual psyche and the collective unconscious by using the metaphor of waves upon an ocean.

The wave represents the individual. The crest of the wave represents the *conscious mind*, which is the state of normal awareness. From this viewpoint, people see themselves as separate, just as each wave appears separate from other waves.

DR. PETER L. JOHNSTON

The body of the wave represents the *personal unconscious*. This part contains all memories not currently in consciousness. The personal unconscious also controls most bodily functions because most organs function below the level of consciousness. There are more than a thousand biochemical reactions occurring every second, all of which are under the control of the personal unconscious. Even conscious movements involve significant input from the personal unconscious. A man smiling as he lifts a beer to his lips uses a large number of muscles in his face, hand, and arm. Some muscles are contracting while others are relaxing in order to allow the movements to occur. Fortunately, there is no need to exercise any great degree of conscious control to carry out such movements. The simple intention of getting the drink to his mouth and the spontaneous pleasure resulting from it are sufficient to trigger the perfect execution of what is truly a complex manoeuvre.

Freud was the great pioneer in understanding the personal unconscious and its workings. He realised the conscious mind was only the visible component of a much larger entity, but he believed the whole psyche, conscious and unconscious, was still confined to the individual.

Where Jung parted company with Freud was in his introduction of the concept of the *collective unconscious*, which he compared with the ocean. The huge dimension of the ocean was an analogy for the vast expansiveness of the collective unconscious mind. The collective unconscious was the source of consciousness for all that exists. As such, it is analogous with the ocean from which all waves derive their form and energy.

In this oceanic realm of the collective unconscious lay the thought patterns common to all humanity. He called them archetypes because they appear in the myths and legends of many cultures as well as in the dreams of individuals.[2]

In his wave model, there were no fixed boundaries between the conscious, the personal unconscious, and the collective unconscious. All were connected. Knowledge could flow from the unconscious into the conscious mind and back again, which is what happens with memories. The individual also has access to the collective unconscious, which provides archetypal energies, dream symbols, and intuitive information.

This idea of a collective unconscious provided an explanation not only for myths and dreams but also for psychic phenomena that were inexplicable in terms of the old paradigm of separate minds.

The collective unconscious also provided an explanation for coincidences and synchronicities.

Personal anecdote 1

In 1971, ten years before I read anything written by Jung, I had a frightening experience. I was called to see a young woman with upper back pain at her home. When I examined her, I could find no clear cause for her pain. Because I felt sure it was true organic pain, I gave her an injection of pethidine and asked her husband to ring me. He rang an hour later to say the pain had settled and she seemed okay.

Some four hours later, I received another request for a home visit to someone else with back pain. When I arrived, the patient had no pain, and in fact, the call seemed to me a waste of time. However, the second patient lived only a few streets away from the patient I had seen that same morning. So I called again to the first young woman's home. Her husband greeted me at the front door by saying, "I'm glad you've called in. She hasn't had any more pain, but I don't think she looks very well." Indeed, she appeared distinctly unwell. She was an ashen colour. On examination, she was in shock and had an abdomen distended with blood. Although she had not missed a period, she had in fact suffered a ruptured ectopic pregnancy that ultimately required twenty-five pints of blood. I have little doubt she would have died but for the coincidence of the other house call—one I had earlier deemed unnecessary!

Personal anecdote 2

Two years later, when I was still practising obstetrics, another young patient went into labour after a healthy and uneventful pregnancy. I examined her when she came into the hospital and was happy with

DR. PETER L. JOHNSTON

her progress. When I finished consulting at my rooms only three hours later, I planned to go home. However, instead of turning right toward home, I absent-mindedly turned left and found myself heading toward the hospital. Once there, I thought I might as well see how the patient was progressing. The labour ward sister put me in my place with her greeting, "What are you back here for? You were only here a few hours ago. Your patient's obs. (clinical observations) are all okay. If there's anything happening, I'll let you know."

Feeling suitably chastened, I walked into the patient's cubicle and had a chat with her. As I was about to leave, the labour ward sister reappeared and said, "While you're here, you might as well do an internal. I set up a tray (examination tray) for another doctor who hasn't turned up." After a short hesitation, I did examine the patient. It was the only time in my life when I felt a prolapsed umbilical cord. The baby had turned in the womb and was presenting as a breech. In the process, the umbilical cord had slipped through underneath and was being compressed by the baby's descent in the pelvis. Because the umbilical cord carried the oxygenated blood to the baby, the baby's oxygen supply was threatened. Fortunately, the cord was still pulsating, so we had a few minutes to get the baby out into the world, where he could breathe in oxygen. We urgently needed an experienced obstetrician. I started by ringing my partner, Rex, who was a general practitioner with considerable obstetric experience. He just happened to be visiting a patient only a few doors from the hospital, and our staff was able to contact him on their first attempt. Within the ten minutes it took me to anaesthetise the patient, Rex was in the labour ward, scrubbed and ready. He performed a rapid and skilled breech extraction, resulting in the birth of a healthy baby.

Personal anecdote 3

When my first wife, Nikki, died in 1987, I wanted her to have a dignified funeral but had no idea where to start. Practical organisational skills are not my forte at the best of times. And this was certainly not the best of times. I had been an emotional wreck for twenty-four hours, totally incapable of organising anything. On the second day of mourning, I had found a sense of inner peace and was ready to see friends who came to our home to share their condolences.

What amazed me was the order in which they arrived. Nikki and I had both been reared as Catholics but had not attended church for some years. Our first visitor was on the local parish committee. One phone call by her and the funeral was booked at our favourite church. The next visitor told us of a celebrant who knew Nikki very well. Another phone call brought an enthusiastic response from the celebrant. The next friend organised appropriate co-celebrants. Then an aunt who was a concert pianist dropped in, offering to play the organ at the local church. My sister arrived soon after. Her connections provided a school choir to accompany the organist. In between visitors, I expressed a wish to have a booklet to accompany the ceremony. Our next visitors were a typist, a calligrapher, and an artist in that order. A brother-in-law who had a new photocopier and the time to copy and collate the booklets arrived after them.

Other visitors suggested hymns that seemed just perfect for the occasion. When we needed readings, I just reached for books in my library, opened them at random, and the perfect words were there on the open pages. Finally, on the night before the funeral, I found myself on my own for the first time in four days. I had the urge to write. For three hours, words for a eulogy flowed in ways I had never experienced before. The string of coincidences made it seem as though an invisible choreographer was orchestrating the whole funeral.

Evaluation

In the foregoing series of personal events, the coincidences were all related to a psychic event—intention. My intention was to help the two patients, but in both cases, there was vital information missing. Coincidences enabled the vital information to be disclosed. In the case of the woman in labour, a coincidence also provided the solution. Looking back on the case of the woman in labour, there were a number of coincidences:

- A decision by my subconscious mind to attend the hospital, which seemed to gain priority over my conscious decision to go home.
- An examination tray set up for another doctor.
- The failure of the other doctor to attend the hospital.
- The labour ward sister's idea and suggestion for me to do an internal examination on the patient.
- My agreement to do so, even when I thought it might have been unnecessary and invasive.
- The ready availability of the obstetrician within minutes.
- No communication delays with the obstetrician, which was crucial when every second counted. In those days before mobile phones, this degree of efficiency was not the norm.

If any one of these seven events had not occurred, I may have delivered a stillborn baby and never have known why.

While mainstream psychiatry has no explanation for synchronicities, Jung's concept of the *collective unconscious* does provide a framework for understanding. The collective unconscious postulates the existence of one consciousness only, with individual minds taking their thoughts from this unitary source. Such a mind would not only be aware of my intentions, the collective mind would have the capacity to implant ideas in the minds of the patient with the mild back pain, the doctor who failed to arrive, the labour ward sister, as well as all the mourners who arrived at our home with their gifts of compassion and organisation.

Transpersonal Psychology

The split between Freud and Jung has continued with their successors. Freud is the father of mainstream psychiatry and psychology. Although most psychiatrists no longer follow Freud's recommendations, they do see each individual psyche as separate. Jung is seen as the father of holistic psychology, which is now called *transpersonal psychology*.

Transpersonal psychology was the outcome of a meeting between Abraham Maslow, a founding father of humanistic psychology, and Stanislav Grof, a psychiatrist with vast experience of altered states of consciousness.

The contribution of Abraham Maslow

Abraham Maslow was a psychologist and philosopher whose interest was human nature in its normal and advanced states of being rather than in diseased states. *Maslow's triangle* postulated that each person has a hierarchy of needs of which food, clothing, and shelter are the most basic. When these basic physical needs are satisfied, emotional and mental needs like love, respect, and self-esteem need to be met. Higher needs are *self-actualisation,* referring to the fulfilment of one's potential, and *transcendence*, meaning spiritual fulfilment and integration of the Self. Maslow believed that full health involved the satisfaction of people's highest psychological needs, including a sense of meaning and an integration of the person.

Transcendence
Self-Actualisation
Self-Esteem, Achievements
Emotional Needs—Love and Belonging
Need for Safety and Security—Physically
Physiological Needs—Food, Clothing, and Shelter[3,4]

Maslow's ideas on psychological health will be discussed further in chapter seventeen.

The contribution of Stan Grof

Stanislav Grof was drawn to a career in psychiatry after he read Sigmund Freud's book titled *The Interpretation of Dreams*. While he was impressed with Freudian theory, he became disillusioned with the tardy and unspectacular results of psychoanalysis. When psychedelic drugs first became available for psychiatric research, Grof offered to trial them. His first experience with psychedelics took him out of his body—and then out of Vienna, Austria, Europe, and finally the earth. This experience changed his life. Thereafter, he devoted his life to understanding what he called "*non-ordinary states of consciousness.*" He induced these states in thousands of clients over a period of thirty years. Initially, he used lysergic acid (LSD) and other hallucinatory drugs. Later, he found he could bring about similar altered states of consciousness without drugs by using a combination of breathing, music, and sometimes touch. He called it *holotropic breathwork.* In some ways, it is a rediscovery of the rituals and "trance states" of indigenous tribes.

Out of this vast experience of 'non-ordinary' states of consciousness, it became obvious to him that experiences in childhood alone could not explain many of the emotional and psychological problems of adulthood.

The three categories of transpersonal psychology

Grof described three categories of conscious states experienced by his clients when they entered altered states. The first he called *postnatal.* This category, one shared by mainstream psychology, comprises memories from childhood and thereafter.

The second he called *perinatal* as many clients regressed to their actual birth process. Birth is a life-and-death situation for a baby, and it can be a terrifying experience. Problems in the pregnancy and in either the first, second, or third stages of labour can be mirrored in the psychiatric problems of adulthood. Regressing to one's birth became a popular form of therapy in the 1980s, when it was referred to as '*rebirthing.*'

The third category was called *transpersonal* because many patients experienced states of being beyond the accepted boundaries of personality. Many left their bodies to experience visions of mythological beings or angels. Some entered into the life of plants and animals and seemed to identify with them. I have even heard someone speak of her experience as the consciousness of a rock. Others went further and experienced life as a person in another era. They could describe the country, the dress, and the buildings of the age to which they regressed. While in the experience, some even spoke in ancient languages. Some travelled to other-worldly places—others to planets or stars where they conversed with extraterrestrials.[5]

Personal Anecdote

With my partner, Jan, we joined a guided tour of Central Australia in 2000. We struck up a friendship with Tim, a young Caucasian man working with a pharmaceutical company. When we visited Stanley Gorge, Tim found a fissure in the rock face, directed his didgeridoo there, and played. The result was awesome. The sound echoed around the canyon. I have heard a number of people, indigenous and Caucasian, play this instrument but none better than Tim. I felt transported to another world. At Gosse's Bluff, the site of an aboriginal massacre, Tim felt the urge to play again. The dirge-like sounds emanating from the didgeridoo brought tears to the eyes of almost all the group.

One night when we were sleeping in swags on a grassy slope in Alice Springs, Tim came to us complaining of severe abdominal pain, as we were the only medical personnel in the group of sixty. However, as tourists, we had no medical equipment, medications, or even a prescription pad. On examination, he was tender over the whole abdomen. While I felt reasonably confident he did not have appendicitis, I really wasn't sure what was causing his pain. He was nauseated but had no other symptoms of gastroenteritis. While I was still trying to think of ways of getting him to the hospital for assessment, Jan worked on reducing his pain by getting him to focus on his breath.

Jan was an experienced nurse who also had knowledge and experience of breathwork. Tim, being skilled with a wind instrument, was able to follow Jan's advice to breathe deeply and in circular fashion, which meant leaving no space between the in and out breaths. After about ten minutes of circular breathing, he stopped writhing and was clearly in an altered state of consciousness. When Jan asked him where he was, he replied, "I am an aborigine. I'm in a settlement somewhere in a dry area of Australia. I have just met a white man, and by his dress, I'd say it's the mid-nineteenth century. I am interested to meet him." Suddenly, Tim clutched his stomach and cried, "He's shot me! Why? I've done nothing to him." He then rolled around in agony for what seemed like a long time but was actually only about twenty seconds according to Jan. Then he lay still in what looked like a light sleep for half an hour—the phase of breathwork called 'integration.'

When he came out of it, he shared with us what for him were new understandings. Firstly, he had died in that lifetime at the hands of a white man who was acting in fear—a fear based in ignorance of the nature of the indigenous Australian. Secondly, he understood his fascination for the indigenous culture. Thirdly, he felt that perhaps a major role in his life would be to help bridge the gap between the white and the black in this country. Finally, he realized that there was more knowledge and wisdom within than he had ever realized before. His pain was gone when he came out of integration, and after he shared his realizations, he gave us both a hug and went back to his own swag. The next morning, he felt great and had no further pain for the remainder of the tour.

Cosmic consciousness

Others had experiences with breathwork so profound they could not describe them. As there seems to be no limit to these experiences, the concept of a universal mind or collective unconscious—one that is unlimited in time and space—made sense to them. Some fortunate clients underwent identification with the Universal Mind. Such experiences have been described in religious scriptures and esoteric texts. The identification with the collective has been described as an experience of *cosmic consciousness*. Such experiences inevitably produce profound changes in these people, but they are not able to articulate the experience in ways that others will understand. Such knowledge is beyond words—the experience is truly out of this world. Parallels may be drawn between the Collective Unconscious, the Universal Mind, and the concept of an infinite God. Because everything originates from thought, the Universal Mind can be seen as the source of all creation. Jung saw the individual psyche as one with it. In his wave analogy, there were no clear boundaries between the conscious and unconscious minds—or between the personal and collective unconscious.

In other words, he saw no separation between the mind of man and the mind of God—not that he made a habit of speaking about God. However, I suspect he might have had an experience of cosmic consciousness. In an interview in the early days of black-and-white television, he was asked if he believed in God. He said that he not so much believed in God but that it was more like he "knew" God. In his autobiography, he described a near-death experience following a heart attack and said this about it: *"What happens after death is so unspeakably glorious that our imaginations and our feelings do not suffice to form even an approximate conception of it."*[6]

Therapies Tapping into the Collective Unconscious

The concept of a collective unconscious suggests the existence of consciousness in all of creation. Plants, animals, and humans all must have consciousness at some level. Bruce Lipton, a prominent molecular biologist, noted that even the simplest life form, the single celled prokaryote, which has no nucleus or mitochondria, demonstrates remarkable intelligence in its capacity for protecting and nurturing itself. It moves towards nurturing environments and away from hostile ones—and opens its membranes to beneficial energies while closing off to toxic ones. In his groundbreaking work, *The Biology of Belief,* he states that *"even though humans are made up of trillions of cells, there is not one new function in our bodies not already expressed in the single cell. That like humans, single cells analysed thousands of stimuli from the microenvironment and select ones appropriate to their survival and growth.*[7]

Jacob Boehme, a sixteenth-century mystic, said that he could look at a growing plant and that by desiring to connect with it, he could enter into the life of the plant, share its ambition to move toward the light, and feel the joy and simplicity of the plant's life.[8] The collective unconscious had an intuitive appeal to me. It seemed to make sense at some deep level, but participating in three forms of psychotherapy brought a more tangible experience of this. These therapies certainly stretched my limits of credibility.

1. Voice Dialogue

In October 1995, I took time off work because of chronic fatigue. Despite some reservations about my energy levels, I attended a four-day conference at Melbourne University because I wanted to hear about the work of Hal and Sidra Stone. Both were Jungian psycho-therapists who had discovered a means of communicating with the archetypes within each individual—a technique they called 'Voice Dialogue.' Their presentation was memorable, not just for the content but for the seamless way in which their words flowed in concert with the audience and with each other.

When Hal called for a volunteer to demonstrate Voice Dialogue, I raised my hand. He asked me to sit opposite him and then asked the others in the group to stand behind me and observe. After a brief chat, he asked permission to speak to my *responsible self*. He then invited me to move my chair to a position where my responsible self would feel comfortable. When I moved my chair to the right, Hal asked me, "How long have you been in Peter's life?" I found myself answering his questions as though I were no longer Peter but only the responsible aspect of Peter.

I spoke about my part in Peter's life and how my role increased when he graduated in medicine, married, and started a family. I was proud of the extent to which I had pushed Peter into becoming a responsible husband, father, family doctor, financier, and health freak. I was even pushing him to play responsible golf! By the time I had finished talking and returned to being Peter again, I was exhausted, and so were many of the onlookers. Hal asked for my permission to interview Peter's *irresponsible self* and invited me to return to Peter.

When I returned my chair to its original position, Hal asked me to find a comfortable place for my irresponsible self. I had been criticised for my laziness for years and had become comfortable with being called lazy. But irresponsibility was something I could never condone in myself. Sensing my discomfort, Hal suggested I take my time and see if I could get in touch with what he described as a clearly *disowned self.* After what seemed a lengthy silence, I yielded to an irresistible urge to throw myself onto the lawn and lie there. Onlookers told me later that I spent much of the time picking little white flowers out of the lawn and throwing them over my shoulder, but I was not conscious of doing so at the time.

What then came forth were recollections of childhood games and irresponsible, enjoyable escapades from university days. Speaking as my irresponsible self, I bemoaned the lack of opportunity for expression in Peter's life. Apart from playing with his four-year-old daughter, the only time I was playing a significant role in Peter's life was when he drank to excess with his old friends—and those times were all too infrequent.

When I returned to my chair and resumed being Peter, Hal asked how I felt energetically. I was amazed. I felt more alive and energetic than I had felt for months. Suddenly, I became aware that my energy had not totally deserted me. It was still there but had been locked away inside. Having been on a stringent diet, exercise, and meditation regime, my direction took an immediate about-turn. With holidays, golf, and a return to a more relaxed regime of eating and drinking, my health improved. While I still advocate a healthy diet, this experience was a very good lesson in balance.

2. Body dialogue

A few months later while I was completing a course in voice dialogue, I learned Hal Stone's daughter, Judith, had initiated a technique called 'body dialogue,' wherein one could gain information by addressing an organ or body part. I struck a credibility problem with this. It seemed to be too far-fetched. I was comfortable with the understanding of consciousness existing everywhere—including a capacity to send our own consciousness anywhere. Yet in practice, I found it difficult to accept the concept of hugging trees and communicating with flowers. Talking to body parts seemed even flakier. What would people think?

At the body dialogue workshop, I drew James as a partner. He, too, was a doctor with an interest in holistic counselling. Though he also had his reservations, he was happy to enter into this 'role play.' Because he had a long and frustrating history of hoarseness, he was happy for me to chat to his larynx. James, then aged sixty-seven, had always been a sensitive man with an interest in music, singing, and art. Speaking informally beforehand, he had told me of his fear-laden, suppressed childhood in an authoritarian, sport-oriented school where corporal punishment was applied lavishly. He had wanted to express his unhappiness at the time but was afraid to do so. He was even afraid of his fear because he could be punished for looking fearful.

He visualised himself shrinking and travelling down to his larynx and merging with it. I was amazed to hear James speak as though he were purely his voice box. His voice box spoke of the struggle. "Inflammatory, rebel-rousing orators, stirring troublemakers, anarchists" were descriptions of the material James was trying to express. As his larynx, he made this statement: "I stop trouble happening by stopping this rebellious energy coming through."

After this dialogue, James realised he had gained a valuable insight. In his work, he had abandoned conventional medicine and was quietly practising holistic psychotherapy in his home. In many ways, he was a rebel, but he feared making waves. He was able to understand how his voice box had become the battleground for this conflict between expressing his truth and staying safe. For the first time, he could see his long-standing laryngitis as an inner conflict.

3.   Sandplay and Gestalt

In 2005, at a workshop studying *sandplay*, participants were asked to put their hands in a sandbox, feel the sand, and move it according to their feelings. They were then invited to choose symbolic objects and place them in the sandbox. They chose from shelves laden with images of insects, trees, vegetation, animals, birds, vehicles, Disney characters, religious figures, and architectural structures. Over five days, I watched and participated in a number of these sandplays. All partic-

THE EAGLE'S WAY

ipants moved the sand, chose their symbols, and placed them in the sand according to what appealed to them at the time. It was not at all cognitive. It was purely intuitive. Yet when the images were arranged, every participant knew they represented an aspect of their lives.

Once they had arranged all their symbols in the sand, a facilitator would ask them to pick up one of their chosen pieces. The facilitator would then ask the client to become the symbol, a process called *gestalt*. While it is like a role-playing exercise, the results were extraordinary. When they had finished the gestalt procedure, each client had gained useful insights into their own lives.

Just as actors can enter into the personality of the characters they are portraying, people seem to be able to enter into the characteristics of the symbol they have chosen. When they speak from the symbol, they bring forward information from the unconscious, which is almost invariably beneficial to their health and well-being.

Summary

Because gestalt can be practised on any symbol or archetype from a rock to a goddess, it appears that people can enter into the consciousness of almost anything. The journey through altered states of consciousness, dream interpretation, gestalt, voice dialogue, and body dialogue seems to allow access to the archetypal energies of the collective unconscious. From the tiny cellular components of organic matter up to the highest cosmic consciousness, anything seems possible.

In using these modalities, I was amazed at the outcomes. These psycho-spiritual technologies brought such frequent synchronicities as to lead me to believe there must be an inner world ready and willing to help people on their journey of self-discovery. When a great teacher said; *"Ask and you will receive; seek and you will find; knock and the door will be opened to you,"* perhaps he was referring to the inner journey?[9]

CHAPTER 8

The New Paradigm Of Mind And Matter

The prevailing scientific view of matter at the beginning of the twentieth century was that all matter was comprised of separate building blocks called atoms. These atoms acted and reacted like sticky billiard balls coming together to form chemical compounds. These atoms would be knocked off their alliances by other chemicals. They would then float free before they recombined with other atoms to form a new chemical compound.

The Quantum Physicist's View of Matter

When it was discovered that there were smaller particles than atoms, these subatomic particles became the new basic particles. This discovery did however undermine the pre-existing common-sense view of matter because it was found that the atom was predominantly open space. Rather like a mini solar system, electrons travelled in an orbit around a central nucleus. However, the size of the particles was incredibly small. The nucleus was about the size of a grain of sand in an atom the size of the Melbourne Cricket Ground. The electrons were so small they could barely be seen unless a spectator had a microscope on hand. Even something as solid as a rock turns out to be more than 99 per cent empty space.

THE EAGLE'S WAY

Further research found little evidence of any solid matter at all in these subatomic particles. They seemed more and more elusive. The positions of subatomic particles were described in terms of probabilities rather than any definite structure. The subatomic particles turned out to be more idealisations than solid particles.[1] According to Niels Bohr, one of the great pioneers of nuclear physics, *"Isolated material particles are abstractions, their properties being definable and observable only through their interactions with other systems."*[2]

Subatomic particles seemed contradictory in nature. Depending on the observer, they could appear as waves at one time and particles at another time. Ultimately, matter was found to be energy—and particles to be very rapidly vibrating pockets of energy. The apparent solidity of matter owes more to its dynamic movement in much the same way a rotating electric fan appears to be a solid disc.

Einstein gave this a mathematical relationship in his famous equation: $e = mc^2$. E was the symbol for energy. m represented matter, and c represented the speed of light. As the speed of light is a constant, this equation equated matter with energy.

Hence, the basic and fundamental substrate of matter has changed from being separate particles to becoming the quantum field of energy, a continuous medium present everywhere in space. Subatomic particles are merely local condensations of this field—concentrations of energy that come and go. Once that concentration disperses, the individual character of the particle disappears and dissolves into the underlying field. As Albert Einstein said, *"We may therefore regard matter as being constituted by the regions of space in which the field is extremely intense. There is no place in this new kind of physics for both the field and matter, for the field is the only reality.*[3]

Instead of a world of separate objects, the familiar world of our senses, the nuclear physicists had substituted an infinite network of interconnecting energies. In the 1930s, when this new view was unfolding, Sir James Jeans, a world-renowned physicist and astronomer, made this comment: *"Today there is a wide measure of agreement that the stream of knowledge is heading towards a non-mechanical reality. The universe begins to look like a great thought rather than like a great machine."*[4]

119

Here is the paradox that relativity and nuclear physics have brought. The absolute truth as seen by physicists is that "all is one." Infinite energy is all there is. It is not unlike the view of our earth the cosmonauts saw from outer space. The vista from there revealed one cohesive planet—only unity and oneness. But in the relative world of our senses, everything appears separate.

Erwin Schrödinger (1887-1961), an Austrian physicist, received the Nobel Prize in 1933 for his contributions to quantum physics. He also made a link between quantum physics and the collective unconscious. He speculated that individual consciousness might only be a manifestation of a unitary consciousness pervading the universe. He used these words: *"Mind, by its very nature, is a singulare tantum. I should say: the overall number of minds is just one."*[5]

The Mind-Body Connection

Nuclear physicists discovered something else quite unexpected when they explored the subatomic world. If a scientist expected a subatomic particle to travel in a certain direction and at a certain speed, it tended to do so. But the same subatomic particles might behave differently for a different experimenter. At this subatomic level, the detached, impartial observer so essential to the scientific method, became impossible. The observer could not just observe subatomic particle movement without in some way affecting the outcome. Fritjof Capra, a nuclear physicist and author of the *Tao of Physics*, wrote this about quantum theory:

> *The crucial feature of quantum theory is that the observer is not only necessary to observe the properties of an atomic phenomenon, but is actually necessary to bring about these properties. If we ask a particle question, we will get a particle answer. If we ask a wave question, we will get a wave answer. The electron does not have objective properties independent of our minds. Hence in atomic physics, the sharp Cartesian division*

between mind and matter and between the observer and the observed can no longer be maintained.[6]

The fact that all the properties of particles are determined by principles, closely related to the methods of observation, would mean that the basic structures of the material world are determined by the way we look at the world. That the observed patterns of matter are reflections of patterns of mind.[7]

Perhaps the authors of the Talmud were onto something when they said *'we see things not as they are but as we are'.*

Dowsing

In the early eighties, I attended a workshop on dowsing and watched people use wire rods to detect underground water. What was of more interest to me was the pendulum. A pendulum is usually a gemstone attached to the end of a chain. All participants were given a pendulum and then told to hold it still above their palms and ask themselves a question with a known answer in the affirmative. When I did this, my pendulum swung back and forth in a vertical axis. Other participants saw their pendulums move in clockwise or anticlockwise directions. Whichever way the pendulum moved, we were told this represented a yes answer to any question. We were then asked to hold the pendulum over the back of our hands and ask a question with a known response in the negative. My pendulum swung back and forth in a horizontal direction, which then became my indicator of a negative response to a question. My fellow students experienced a similar response. Their pendulums swung or rotated in the opposite direction to that of their positive response.

The pendulum provided an example of quantum principles. It moved according to the mental state of the holder. While initially we asked questions with known answers, later the pendulum responded with positive or negative swings to genuine queries—and when our questions lacked clarity the pendulum responded indecisively.

DR. PETER L. JOHNSTON

Applied kinesiology

Another modality I came across in the early eighties was *Touch for Health*. It involved measuring muscle strength and vitality and treating the patient with lymphatic massage and meridian therapy. Founded by George Goodheart, a chiropractor, the concept expanded into many areas of health, most of them under the category of kinesiology. The key diagnostic tool was 'muscle testing.' A specific muscle could be used as an 'indicator muscle' to gain information from the subconscious. Like a pendulum, a muscle would give a yes or no answer to a question. The indicator muscle would weaken when the answer was in the negative but would remain firm or become stronger when the answer was affirmative. I have continued to use this technique as an aid in assessing food intolerances and compatibility with medications.

Mind over matter

It is taken as a fact that fire burns. Even if one's attention is elsewhere when an ember flicks out of a fireplace, it burns if it lands on flesh. Yet at a seminar I attended in Sydney in 1995, Anthony Robbins convinced over two thousand attendees that they could walk over a bed of hot coals and not get burned. On that night, more than two thousand of us changed a physical reality by changing our states of consciousness.

This phenomenon has been demonstrated in the medical field too. Hypnosis is an altered state of consciousness where the client is in a more focused and concentrated state of mind. When hypnotherapists have suggested to clients that a cold object was hot, clients have produced blisters on their skin at the site of contact.[8,9]

The body as a servant of consciousness

Severe child abuse can result in a condition known as *multiple personality disorder*. The afflicted child unconsciously tries to escape this unacceptable world by walling off the normal sub-personalities from each other. Hence, it seems as though multiple different personalities live in the same body, each personality unaware of the existence of the others. What has been observed in some of these is that a patient may suffer from asthma or allergies while he or she is operating from one of the personalities but have no problems when he or she is manifesting from another. So, even though these personalities share the same body, because each of them has a different mental and emotional outlook, the body arranges its molecules to fit the personality operating at the time.[10]

While I have had a patient with multiple personality disorder, I have not seen her switch from one personality to another. However, I have seen a young Australian woman act as a trance channel for a disembodied spiritual teacher who was male. She was in her late twenties, quiet and rather shy as she asked those gathered around her to try to be quiet while she entered a trance. Moments later, she stood up and proceeded to speak in a strong voice with a foreign accent and an amusing pronunciation of English words and phrases. Her posture and gait were totally different as were the gestures and the way she addressed each individual. It looked to me like a great acting performance, but when she answered questions for two hours, I realised it was beyond anything any actress could do.

One day, I saw her struggling with a runny nose and a rather hoarse voice. The symptoms ceased while she was channelling but returned when she emerged from her trance. She told us she was allowing a spiritual being to use her body to transmit his teachings. I have no reason to doubt her explanation as I could not come up with any other rational explanation for what I observed. It seemed to be another demonstration of the way the body responds to the consciousness occupying it.

Mind-body disease

Although the mind-body connection had been recognised for years, serious scientific research on the subject only got under way in the mid-twentieth century. Franz Alexander, a Hungarian physician and psychoanalyst, established the Chicago Institute for Psychoanalysis in 1932. For over twenty years, the institute conducted extensive research on emotional disturbance and psychosomatic disease, identifying various disorders with particular unconscious conflicts.[11]

The word *psychosomatic* is derived from the Greek words *psyche,* meaning 'soul,' and *soma,* meaning 'body.' Among the disorders considered to have psychosomatic connections by the medical profession are migraine, asthma, tension headache, peptic ulcer, inflammatory bowel disease, irritable bowel syndrome, impotence, and hypertension.

The role of stress in other chronic diseases, such as heart disease, cancer, and rheumatoid arthritis, has raised questions as to whether the psyche's involvement in disease might be greater than previously thought. Uncontrolled emotional stress was shown statistically to be a more potent factor than smoking in death from cancer and heart disease.[12] Another study of patients with established heart disease showed stress to be the strongest predictor of future heart attacks.[13] Another study involving 1,623 patients who had survived heart attacks found that those who tended to react angrily to unwelcome situations had twice the rate of subsequent heart attacks compared to those who remained calm.[14]

The water connection

Samuel Hahnemann, the founder of homeopathy, was a medical practitioner who restricted its use to qualified medical practitioners. Despite its origins and its use over two hundred years, homeopathy has never been recognised by mainstream medicine because it fails to meet the requirements of science and common sense. Homeopathic remedies are formed by successively diluting active ingredients in water and alcohol, shaking the remedy each time before further dilution. The paradoxical result is that the greater the dilution, the stronger the potency. The highest potencies are so dilute that they have no physical ingredient in the mixture. To conventional science, the high-potency homeopathic was simply a mixture of water and alcohol.

Homeopathic theory postulated a non-physical healing agent—a subtle energy transferred through all dilutions by a shaking process called succussion. Water was considered an appropriate vehicle for this energy, while alcohol helped preserve the energy for a longer period.

Dr. Edward Bach, a prominent bacteriologist and homeopath, took this further when he discovered the capacity of natural flowers and shrubs to provide vibrational healing for mental and emotional states. He also chose water as a vehicle to transmit these healing vibrations to his patients. It was quite a stretch for me to believe in the power of plants to affect human moods and beliefs, let alone the capacity to bottle the power. Yet there was no mistaking their effectiveness in treating the emotional problems of babies and infants. While they worked for me, I was happy to sit with the mystery. In 2005, twenty years after first using flower essences, I heard about the work of Masaru Emoto, which I mentioned previously.

In 1994, with the help of a research assistant, Emoto found a way to freeze water and take microphotographs of it. In his early work, he found natural, untreated water formed crystals, whereas Japanese tap water did not. Soon after, he realised water froze into different shapes according to the information and emotional energy the water received. He started by putting the same water into two glass bottles. On the first, he pasted a label typed "thank you," and on the second, he used a label with "you fool." The water in the first bottle formed beautiful hexagonal crystals while the second showed only crystal fragments. Similar results came using other polarised labels such as "happiness" and "unhappiness," "well done" and "no good," "like" and "dislike," and "power" and "powerless." Gratitude, written in six different languages, consistently resulted in the formation of beautiful crystals.[15] The body is said to be 70 per cent water, although the proportion varies from 88 per cent in babies to around 60 per cent with the desiccation of old age. Perhaps the water content of the body is facilitating the transfer of mental and emotional energies to the physical body.

The mind-to-brain connection

Our ability to understand the brain increased dramatically with the invention of CT and MRI scans. Yet the introduction of micro-mapping has extended this knowledge even further. While this is still mainly used as a research tool, scientists can follow the pathway of an individual nerve cell by working under a microscope with tiny instruments.[16] By using brain-mapping techniques, Alvaro Pascuel-Leone at Harvard Medical School showed that we change the anatomy of our brains simply by using our imagination.[17]

In one experiment, he taught two groups of non-pianists to play a sequence of notes. He asked one group to play the sequence for two hours per day for five days. The other group was asked to sit at the keyboard and imagine playing and listening to the sequence for the same ten hours. He found both groups learned to play the piece and both showed similar changes in their brain maps.[18]

More surprising was a study involving not just brain mapping but physical strength. One group exercised a finger muscle for four weeks. The other group imagined exercising the same finger while they imagined a voice shouting, "Harder, harder, harder." At the end of the four weeks, the exercise group had increased their muscular strength by 30 per cent, but the imagining group had increased theirs by 22 per cent, no doubt because of the increased area of brain tissue related to that finger.[19]

In 2006, a team from Brown University implanted a tiny silicone chip with one hundred electrodes into the brain of a twenty-five-year-old quadriplegic. After four days of practice, the young man was able to move a cursor on a computer screen, adjust the channels on his television, and control a robotic arm, using only thought and intent.[20]

The missing link

In 1972, Candace Pert, a graduate student in neuroscience, created a scientific breakthrough when she discovered the opiate receptor in the brain. Candace assumed the body did not create this receptor just to enjoy drugs derived from poppies. This opened up a new area of research leading to the discovery of the body's natural opiates. Called endorphins, these morphine-like substances not only reduce pain but are also capable of creating a blissful state rather like the one created by heroin.

THE EAGLE'S WAY

In the early eighties, I was encouraging my cancer patients to attend meditation groups. Some of those in chronic pain would find relief during meditation. When I heard Candace speak about endorphins in 1997, I realised those patients might have been tapping into their body's natural pain-relieving chemicals. Perhaps the endorphins were also involved in the 'blissed-out' state achieved by some people in meditation.

Scientists from different fields working on these endorphins discovered that these molecules belong to a class of very small proteins called *peptides* that have been found to regulate moods and emotions. Candace Pert and colleagues mapped peptide receptors and found dense clusters of them in parts of the brain associated with emotion. She also found them in areas of the brain associated with memory. Even more interesting, peptide networks were found throughout the body in organs, glands, and tissues.[21]

She refers to the peptides as the "*biochemical correlates of emotion*" and believes emotional memory is stored throughout the body.[22] She also came to a very interesting conclusion about the relationship between the mind and the body. Her research suggested that it was not so much the power of mind over matter. In terms of human physiology, the mind becomes the body. She saw the body and mind as one.[23]

Cellular memory

In the early eighties, I met Bob, a radiographer who was changing careers. He had become very interested in postural integration, a form of deep tissue massage. When he worked on deep fascia, it was not uncommon for his clients to experience profound emotions and recall traumatic experiences from their childhood. We met at a counselling workshop. Bob was attending because he needed to develop skills to deal with his clients' experiences. Later, when I was learning another form of energy massage called Bowen therapy, I observed clients going into emotional states in much the same way Bob had described.

In 1997, I heard Candace Pert and her husband, Michael Ruff, a virologist, speak about emotions in the form of peptides being

DR. PETER L. JOHNSTON

located throughout the body. When they mentioned energy being held in packets in the tissues, it all started to make sense. Perhaps the unexpressed emotions of past events could be locked up in the tissues. When a person sought help and a therapist touched into those deeper areas, whether physically or energetically, the emotions and memory of the event were being released.

Paul Pearsall, a psychoneuroimmunologist, had a bone marrow transplant for cancer that led to a deep interest in the lives of transplant donors and recipients. His research left him convinced of the capacity for the heart to not only retain memory but also carry a code representing the soul, which would be transmitted to every cell in the body. Some heart-transplant recipients showed interesting changes in their personalities, food preferences, and attitudes. Their new qualities were similar to those of their donors.

While Paul was addressing a group of psychotherapists, a psychiatrist came to the microphone and shared an extraordinary story. Sobbing to the extent that the audience had difficulty understanding her words, she spoke about an eight-year-old girl who received the heart of a ten-year-old. The mother brought the child to the psychiatrist because the little one was having nightmares about a man who had killed her donor. After several sessions, the psychiatrist could not deny the child's story. As a result, the psychiatrist and the child's mother contacted the police. The police apprehended the murderer, who was convicted on the evidence provided by the young girl. The site and time of the crime, the clothes he wore, and the words the victim spoke before her death were all found to be completely accurate.[24]

The physiology of experience

Neuropeptide receptors are located almost entirely in the sensory or incoming areas of the nervous system. The visual pathway is especially refined, having six synapses between the retina and the visual cortex of the brain. All these synapses are storage sites for visual memories, meaning that all visual experiences are being filtered through areas containing data from the past. To a lesser extent, this is happening throughout the body, as peptides exist in all parts of the body, especially those areas processing information. This remarkably complex system has the capacity to suppress, exaggerate, or distort the incoming data according to the beliefs, interests, and desires of the individual.[25]

In summary

I refer to the peptides as the missing link because they link the physical body with the mind. While Candace Pert calls peptides *"the molecules of emotion,"* emotions are usually a human response to experience and belief. Cellular memories are not only pockets of emotion—they are memories of experiences. In this sense, the peptides link the body to thoughts, beliefs, emotions, and experiences. They provide the best scientific evidence of the mechanism by which the mind speaks to the body. Candace sees the body as an extension of the mind—a *"body-mind."* Thoughts and feelings translate into peptides. Thoughts and words become flesh.

Far from the mind and body being separate, the new paradigm reveals an intricate connection between the intellect, emotions, and memories with the nervous system, endocrine system, and immune system.

The Ecological View

Until the mid-twentieth century, biologists were occupied in studying the nature of individual plants and animals and their evolutionary aspects. In the late nineteenth century, there was some scientific approach to ecology but not in any depth. In 1946, serious study of the ecosystem was initiated, and a new understanding of the interconnectedness of life began to unfold.

The principles underlying the study of ecosystems are based on the view that all the elements of a life-supporting environment of any size, whether natural or man-made, are parts of an integral network in which each element interacts directly or indirectly with all others and affects the function of the whole. All ecosystems are contained within the largest, the ecosphere that encompasses the entire physical earth and all of its biological components.

Systems ecology has also given another wonderful example of the paradox of relative separation but overall oneness. Each plant, animal, mineral, inorganic substance, and human is unique and individual. Yet at the same time, there is a constantly changing energy in the unity of the one energy—the ecosphere.

The Rise of Holism

Putting a man on the moon is often quoted as the pinnacle of scientific and technological achievement. Yet when Neil Armstrong took his "giant step for mankind" in 1969, mankind was starting to shift away from the successful analytical approach that took us to the moon. The shift was toward an integrative holistic perspective.

Holism or *wholism* can be summed up in one sentence: *The whole is greater than the sum of the parts.* To understand this concept, it is necessary to understand its opposite—*reductionism*. Reductionism is the belief that entities are collections of more simple entities. A living cell is a collection of molecules. A human body is a collection of cells. This reduction of life to its basic building blocks has been an important part of the scientific paradigm, and much of medical science is built around it. The division of our medical expertise into specialists treating separate organs and systems recognises this reductionist attitude.

While the reductionist view is true, the holistic view is that the whole person is much more than the sum total of his or her organs, systems, and cells. Amoebae, which are single-celled organisms, may accumulate in large numbers, but their level of function as a group will not match that of the same number of cells combined to form a multi-cellular organism such as an ant. In other words, an ant as a whole organism is more than just a combination of cells. Similarly, a colony of ants acting in the coordinated way it normally does, functions at a higher level than the same number of ants acting individually.

In human physiology, clusters of cells function at a more differentiated level when they become glands, while glands are more effective combined and integrated into organs such as the pancreas. A unified team can achieve more than the players can individually. A rowing eight can go faster than eight single scullers. A unified nation is a stronger force than its individual population.

Holism and humanistic psychology

Holistic medicine is a product of this viewpoint, seeing human beings as more than just the sum of their parts. The holistic approach is to treat body, mind, emotions, and spirit as all being part of an indivisible whole. Unlike conventional Western medicine that uses analysis, holistic medicine employs synthesis.

While it draws from many sources, there is little doubt humanistic psychology played a significant part in the holistic approach to health care. The humanistic movement developed in the 1950s as an alternative to behavioural therapy and psychoanalysis, which were the dominant schools of psychology at that time. Both were analytical in nature. Both saw human behaviour as resulting from conditioning or events in childhood, both of which rendered the behaviour difficult to change. The first of five basic postulates of the Association for Humanistic Psychology states, *"Man, as man, supersedes the sum of his parts."*[26]

While Maslow and Carl Rogers were the major pioneers of the humanistic approach, I was most impressed by a little book called *Man's Search for Meaning.* Dr. Victor Frankl, a Jewish neurologist from Vienna, survived four German concentration camps. The great gem he extracted from the Holocaust was the power of meaning to sustain life. He observed that once people lost hope, they soon died. Those for whom life had lost its meaning frequently died before they even reached the gas chambers. Yet those who found a purpose could maintain their mental health in the most appalling physical and mental conditions imaginable. The camps were places where every attempt was made to strip away any vestige of self-esteem a prisoner might gather. The capacity of these people to change and

The Concept of the Hologram

Traditional understanding of the relationship between wholes and parts has always been quite simple. Wholes contain parts. Parts make up the whole. However, from another aspect, it could be seen differently. The body as a whole is made up of billions of cells. Yet the whole body develops from one cell. The original fertilised egg cell contains the blueprint for the whole body in much the same way an acorn carries the blueprint for the oak tree.

In 1948, Dennis Gabor, a Hungarian-born scientist, introduced the concept of holography, for which he was awarded the Nobel Prize in 1971. However, until the development of lasers in the early sixties it was not possible to produce these three-dimensional images in two-dimensional formats.

When a true hologram is cut into pieces, an unusual thing occurs. Each part carries an image of the whole picture. The original image appears on each fragment. This does not happen to the holographic images on credit cards and some art, which are not true holograms.

Holography in health

The discovery of the DNA molecule by Watson and Crick in 1953 unveiled a biochemical marvel. Here was the whole genetic code, so many individual human characteristics, all carried on a double helix molecule in each cell of the body. And all of this information was being transmitted faithfully to each succeeding generation of cells. Each tiny particle of the body was carrying the blueprint of the whole. Here, in biology, was the same holographic principle.

At the macroscopic level, there are some interesting parallels too. An iridologist views the iris as a map of the whole body, revealing the functional states of its organs and systems. Reflexologists see the

THE EAGLE'S WAY

bodily organs mapped out on the feet. Practitioners of aural acupuncture see the body drawn upside down on the outer ears of their clients. Practitioners of the ancient art of palmistry see the life of a client laid out in the palm of his or her hand. I have experienced an intuitive diagnostician reel off much of my life history just by holding my right foot. In all these modalities, the whole appears in the part.

When people are healthy, their cells work together very well, presumably aided by the knowledge that each cell carries the template for the whole body. And when people are unwell, organs compensate for each other, suggesting there are very effective information networks between organs and their cellular components.

Karl Pribram, an eminent neurophysiologist from Stanton University, was puzzled by a colleague's failure to demonstrate specific sites in the brain where memories were stored. In the 1940s, he concluded memories were not limited to one area of the brain but were stored throughout the brain. However, he had no idea of the mechanism until he read about holograms in 1966. When he heard of the enormous storage capacity of holograms and the way they worked, he saw this holographic model as the best way of explaining the brain's ability to store memory and its capacity to recall and forget memories, to project images, and to experience flashbacks.[28]

Is the universe holographic?

Albert Einstein broke new ground when he saw time and space not as separate entities but as a time-space continuum. David Bohm, a nuclear physicist who worked with Einstein at Princeton, went a step further in postulating the whole universe, from consciousness to matter, as being a continuum. He saw all visible life and matter as the *explicate* or *unfolded* aspect of an invisible, constantly changing, undivided whole. He referred to this undivided whole as the *implicate* or *enfolded* order. In Bohm's view of the universe, what we perceive to be reality is actually a projected holographic image. He saw the whole cosmos as a hologram.[29]

Philosophers have wondered whether our universe is a hologram. Could we, as individuals, carry the blueprint for the cosmos in the same way our cells carry it for the whole person? Are people unconsciously carrying vast knowledge of the universe, but are only some like Einstein able to tap into this? Are people who have experiences of 'cosmic consciousness' experiencing this but unable to explain it with the limits of language? Whether there is any validity in any of this speculation, the hologram does at least provide an interesting metaphor for the relationship between our individual selves and the universe as a whole. Deeper truths, which are difficult to express and understand in scientific terms, can find expression in the language of poetry. Maybe the English poet William Blake (1757-1827) might have glimpsed the new paradigm a hundred years earlier when he wrote these lines:

> To see a world in a grain of sand,
> And a heaven in a wild flower,
> Hold infinity in the palm of your hand,
> And eternity in an hour . . .
> We are led to believe a lie
> When we see with, not thro' the eye.
> Which was born in a night, to perish in a night.
> When the soul slept in beams of light.[30]

CHAPTER 9

The Re-Emergence Of Ancient Wisdom

The new paradigm highlights an existential paradox. Science, psychology, and ecology are demonstrating the unity of existence. On the other hand, our intellect and senses remind us of our separation. While the new paradigm might have brought this paradox into prominence, it is by no means new. Humanity has been grappling with this paradox for a long time.

The Search for Truth in the West

Projection is a phenomenon described by Sigmund Freud as an ego-defence mechanism. As mentioned previously, projection is actually an unconscious, automatic process in all perception. In the everyday observation of material objects like chairs and stoves, there may be little difference between individual perceptions. However, something emotional, dramatic, or controversial may provide many different versions of the same event from different observers.

The search for objective truth in the Western world led to the jury system and the scientific method. Because larger numbers reduce the significance of each individual's unique view, they increase the likelihood of acquiring a more objective version of the facts.

Plato was suspicious of the senses because they could be so easily deceived. Conjurers know "the hand is quicker than the eye" and make a living demonstrating their capacity to trick the viewer. Plato, while not ignoring input from the senses, believed one had to go beyond the senses to find truth. Other philosophers, including Descartes, have tended to agree. The great Christian philosophers Augustine and Thomas Aquinas integrated the philosophies of Plato and Aristotle and attempted to prove the existence of God as the creative force of life.

Two thousand years after Plato, Immanuel Kant proposed that everything we apprehend comes via the nervous system and five senses. Given the limitation of our senses, this puts a significant limit on our ability to find ultimate truth. Since Kant, most philosophers and scientists have accepted the existence of God to be something that can neither be proven nor disproved.[1]

The current thinking in conventional science appears to be that the universe is continuing to expand since the big bang and that environmental pressure and natural selection have, by a random process, produced the remarkably complex world we live in. Stephen Hawking, the renowned physicist, suggests the existence of God is unnecessary to explain the origin of the universe.[2] Richard Dawkins, a leading biologist, sold over two million copies of his book titled *The God Delusion,* contending that a supernatural creator almost certainly does not exist.[3]

In contrast, Einstein was said to be spiritually aligned with the philosophy of Benedict Spinoza (1632-67).[4] Spinoza believed God to be inclusive of all thought and matter—that God is the world and not separate from it.[5] Einstein has been quoted as making these statements.

- My religion consists of a humble admiration of the illimitable superior spirit who reveals himself in the slight details we can perceive with our frail and feeble mind.[6]
- I am convinced that He (God) does not play dice.[7]
- A human being is a part of a whole, called by us 'universe,' a part limited in time and space. He experiences himself,

his thoughts and feelings, as something separated from the rest—a kind of optical illusion of his consciousness.[8]

Leonard Mlodinow, a prominent scientist and co-author with Stephen Hawking of *The Grand Design,* describes consciousness as *"science's last frontier"* and writes that *in 2010, science does not even have a good operational definition of it.*[9] So what follows could be described as 'complementary or alternative' science.

The Search for Truth in the East

Eastern philosophers, mystics, and sages have also questioned the accuracy of the senses but have been equally suspicious of the mind. They have viewed the intellect not only as the assessor, classifier, and judge of the sensory data but also as the unconscious distorter of the sensory input.

Because we project our own mental concepts onto what our eyes perceive, we actually see with our minds as well as our eyes. The same phenomenon seems to occur with our other senses too. All of our senses detect vibrations within a certain range and send these messages to the nervous system, which interprets them and responds accordingly. All of this is done instantaneously and subconsciously. This means that all we ever know is what our own minds bring to us. Every human experience of the physical world is mentally interpreted and hence subjective.

Perhaps this is why the Hindus refer to this material world as *maya,* meaning illusion. The well-known Eastern fable of the six blind men and the elephant has various translations but goes like this: One holds a leg and thinks it's a tree trunk. Another holds a tusk and thinks it's a pipe. Another holds the trunk and thinks it is a snake. While others thinks the tail is a rope, the flank is a wall, and an ear is a fan. Yet there is a deeper symbolic meaning underlying the story. The six blind men represent the five senses and the intellect, while the elephant represents Brahman, the truth of all that exists. The limitations of the intellect and sensory perceptions do not allow comprehension of ultimate truth. Yet that truth is there awaiting a different type of vision.

This different vision is about looking inside rather than out. To use an analogy, an amateur astronomer who does not know the features and limitations of his telescope might mistake a firefly for a shooting star. Philosophers, like astronomers, need to know the limitations of their instrument. And the instrument used by philosophers is the mind. In order to receive truth, one would need to be aware of the distortions of one's own mind—the beliefs, the expectations, and the prejudices. The search for truth requires much work. The sages of the East were not alone in their focus on self-knowledge. The ancient Greeks had similar ideas. Their Delphic oracle proclaimed, "*Man, know thyself.*"

Looking for the Self

Because personal belief, prejudice, and negative emotional states distort the perception of truth, it makes good sense to clean the windscreen of perceptions by finding and, if possible, removing the elements obscuring the view. However, one major hurdle is the unconscious nature of so many personal beliefs, attitudes, and expectations. An even greater difficulty lies in altering the mind when people believe the mind is their identity. I have heard people say, "That's me—that's the way I've always been. I can't just change myself." How does somebody change their thinking when they believe it is unchangeable?

I, too, believed I was a body controlled by a mind. I assumed my thoughts, beliefs, values, and goals emanated from my brain. Yet at the same time, I was always aware of being the same person. I was forty years of age before I queried this assumption. I asked myself this question: If I am this same continuous self, who am I?[10]

Here is where my assumptions hit a roadblock. Neither my body nor brain could fit the description of a continuous 'same-I entity.' My body at forty was a very different shape than what it was at four. Under a microscope, change is seen to be continuous. Skin cells are constantly dying and being replaced. With sunburn, the cells peel off even faster. Blood cells are replaced approximately every six weeks,

THE EAGLE'S WAY

which allows blood donors to make regular contributions. Organ cells last longer and muscle cells longer still. Nerve cells, including those of the brain, last the longest, but seven years is the estimated average life span of these, according to neurophysiologists. Hence, even our brain cells are undergoing change all the time.

If that unchanging 'I' is not my body, it is obviously not my thoughts or emotions either. My thoughts are constantly changing, and my emotions and moods do likewise.

Could it be my personality? My personality is the side of me I project to the world. Derived from the word *persona,* meaning 'mask,' it does not always represent what I genuinely believe about myself. However, it does not remain static either. My personality is certainly different from what it was when I was a child. It has gradually changed with age and experience. It is certainly not beyond the capacity to regress. When I celebrate with old friends, I can rapidly revert to the habits of my twenties. I notice these personality changes because I am that which does not change and I can observe such fluctuations.

Is my 'ego' my true essence? Ego is the Latin word for 'I' and is what I take myself to be. Unlike my personality, my ego is not just what I show to the world. This is what I actually believe myself to be. Nevertheless, my perception of me keeps changing. My ego can be inflated or wounded according to circumstances. Sometimes this descent from "top cock to feather duster" takes only a minor setback to achieve. Yet there is still an 'I' entity that can observe this changing attitude toward myself. There is a 'same-I entity' behind the 'changing I' of my ego.

When all other options have been eliminated, who else can this 'I-entity' be but *consciousness?* My *un*changing identity must be consciousness.

The Reality of Self

Once I realised my true and unchanging identity was consciousness, it became easier to understand how I could be conscious but separate from my brain and body. When I am dreaming, my consciousness might be in a bus going over a cliff, but my body is in bed, taking a distinctively less active role in the event. While it might be only a dream, it is very real to me while I am in it. I can be just as anxious, if not more so, in a nightmare as I can be in a stressful life event.

A scene from *Monty Python's Flying Circus* showed a man blindfolded and handcuffed to a wooden post. A squad of Latin American soldiers were taking aim at him with rifles. Suddenly, he woke up in bed in a sweat and was very relieved to see his mother there. He exclaimed, "Mother, I have had such an awful nightmare. It's such a relief to be home with you again."

His mother replied, "No dear. This is a dream. You are actually in front of a firing squad in South America!"

Consciousness cannot be observed scientifically as consciousness is the observer. Hence, it remains a mystery—a vast mystery. Nevertheless this great mystery has prompted much searching in many cultures. So it was to spiritual texts I turned, starting with the familiar Judaeo-Christian scriptures.

Scriptural References to Consciousness

From my schooldays, the words *Yahweh* and *Jehovah* were familiar to me as names for the Hebrew God. What surprised me was the discovery of the meaning of these words. They came from the Hebrew word *YHWH*, meaning "I *am* that I *am*":

> *And God said unto to Moses, I AM THAT I AM:*
> *And he said, Thus shalt thou say unto the*
> *children of Israel,*
> *I AM hath sent me unto you.*[11]
> *This is my name forever.*[12]

I can think of no better description of consciousness than the words "I am."

God is described as the creator of all that is—the all-knowing, all-powerful, infinite, loving, eternal presence. If God is truly everywhere, then God must also be present in all beings. God must be the consciousness in all life forms—The *I am* that is *I am* to all that is—

THE EAGLE'S WAY

their consciousness, their awareness, their *life*. After all, the difference between a dead body and a living being is consciousness—life.

Jesus used this name for God in some of his utterances: *"I am the resurrection and the life."*[13] *"I am the way, the truth and the life; no man cometh unto the Father but by me."*[14]

Jesus used the Aramaic word *Abba* to describe consciousness in its universal form. Translated as 'Father,' Jesus used it to differentiate the infinite consciousness from the individual consciousness dwelling within each person. He referred to the latter as the 'son.' He nevertheless made it clear there was but one consciousness: *"The Father and I are one.*[15] *The words I have spoken to you do not come from me. The Father, who remains in me does his own work."*[16] He also made it clear that he was referring to all of humanity when he spoke of the son *"Behold, the kingdom of God is within YOU.*[17] *YE are all gods.*[18] *OUR Father, which art in heaven."*[19]

Christianity declared Jesus to be the only son of God. Perhaps, if his words had been interpreted as representing the life of everybody, what John the evangelist referred to as *"the light that lighteth every man that cometh into the world,"*[20] religious wars on our planet might have been considerably less frequent.

The Islamic *Quran* describes God as being *"nearer to man than the jugular vein."*[21] The Hindu scriptures, the *Upanishads* and the *Bhagavad Gita* describe a similar relationship between the individual and the "Supreme Being" dwelling within in the examples provided:

> *The Self is all-knowing, it is all-understanding, and to it belongs all glory. It is pure consciousness, dwelling in the heart of all, in the divine citadel of Brahma. There is no space it does not fill. Dwelling deep within, it manifests as mind, silently directing the body and the senses. The wise behold this Self, blissful and immortal, shining forth through everything.* (Mundaka Upanishad)

> *Of all that is material and all that is spiritual in this world, know for certain that I AM both its origin and dissolution. The Supreme Lord is situated in everyone's heart, and is directing the wanderings of all living*

*entities. Surrender unto Him utterly—and by His grace you will attain
transcendental peace and the Supreme and eternal abode.* (Bhagavad Gita)

I use the word 'God' in this book because it has been the traditional word used for the creative force of life. Yet, like 'Father,' the word can have negative connotations, so I prefer to avoid both of these words. Because God is used to justify war, persecution, and other unwholesome activities, the word has become debased. Also, there are too many false images of God.

In truth, *all* images of God are false. As the Chinese philosopher Lao-Tze put it in the first three lines of his famous Tao Ching: "*The Tao (Way) that can be spoken is not the eternal Tao. The name that can be named is not the eternal name. The nameless is the origin of Heaven and Earth.*"

The infinite cannot be encapsulated in any image. God is another word for collective or universal consciousness. As such, God is the observer and creator of all that exists. God is also the quantum field of energy, the infinite field of matter. As such, God is the creation and substance of all that exists. The vastness of this is beyond imagination. Childhood images of God as a bearded gentleman organizing earthly affairs from a distant heaven are not helpful—they separate creator from creation. I prefer words like *Consciousness, Life,* or *All that is.* While these words are also incapable of encapsulating the divine, they are at least more generalized, abstract terms. As such, they are harder to concretize into images and forms—and as metaphors for God, they are at least inclusive of humanity.

The Illusory Self

When my daughter Lara was a baby, her grandmother gave her a stuffed toy in the form of a pillow with a dog's face on it. Its official name was Bonzo. It was always with her. She slept with it and carried it everywhere, and when she could speak, she called it Bom. When normal wear and tear required Bom to be washed, Lara would patiently wait under the clothesline for Bom to dry. Over time, the washing eroded the dog's face, so her mother would sew another cover and I would paint Bom's face on it. It did not seem to worry Lara that my drawings of Bom were done faster and less accurately each time we needed to replace it. Eventually, I got so lazy that she was carrying nothing but a little white pillow with no drawing on it and the umpteenth lot of stuffing inside it. Yet to Lara, it was still her beloved Bom. She continued to carry her security companion everywhere despite the fact there was not a single remnant of the original. Bom was really only a mental construction to which Lara was attached.

Maybe our egos are like Bom—mental constructs that arrive in infancy and to which we become attached. When, as infants, we become aware we are no longer part of our mothers, we develop a concept of ourselves as separate beings. We are given an individual name to differentiate us from other people. As our infantile senses become more acute, we can see our obvious physical separation from everybody else. Our identification with our individual bodies is felt more acutely when we are in pain, hunger, or physical discomfort. As we grow and mature, so does the assumption of our separateness. Why would we question what seems so obvious?

Yet the reality of our egos is built on the evidence of our senses, our individual names, our past histories, and our mental pictures of being separate. Experience has shown the senses to be an adequate guide to relative truth but an inaccurate guide to absolute truth. While we speak of some people having 'big egos,' in truth all egos are fragile because they rely on sensory and mental illusion for their survival. Every experience happens in the present moment. The past is just a mental image of a present moment that has passed. The future is a projected mental image. The ego depends on past history and future goals for its identity and existence—yet both are just images. In dementia and amnesia, these images can be lost.

The Inner Path to Self-Realisation

The role of the intellect is to evaluate and make decisions based on choosing from a variety of options. Its role is in the world of separate objects, beings, and experiences. The intellect is indispensable on this three-dimensional planet, but awareness of the unified realm of consciousness requires going beyond this everyday state of mind.

Observing thoughts helps take a person into a state of consciousness. When people can view their thoughts, beliefs, and feelings from a detached and compassionate perspective, they are operating from consciousness. Spiritual texts have referred to this state as *higher consciousness*, which is a more accurate description. Consciousness is present everywhere, including in all intellectual activity, so in truth, nobody is ever completely unconscious—even when asleep or comatose. However, most people identify themselves with their ego-based mind, and hence, they are unaware of the higher dimensions of their reality. By quietly observing the activity of their minds, they enter a different state of awareness. They become the silent witness to the mind. Meditation and contemplation are terms used to describe this process of moving beyond the busy mind.

Meditation is not about stopping mental activity. It is the job of the mind to produce thoughts, and it does its job very well. Forcing it to be quiet does not work. However, closing off from busy intellectual activity is helpful. Observing flowers, candles, or objects of beauty can be used as a means of entering a meditative state. Walking quietly in natural surroundings is a form of contemplation facilitating higher consciousness. Closing one's eyes, directing attention to one's breathing, or listening to silence have long been popular meditative techniques.

Buddhism has always encouraged a state of *mindfulness,* which actually means keeping one's focus in the present time. It means being fully conscious of what one is doing even while one is performing mundane domestic tasks like washing dishes. It can mean being aware of the muscular action of one's tongue and jaw while one is eating breakfast. Not easy to do with a newspaper on the breakfast table!

Contemplative strategies involve relaxation, but also much more. There are many books available on the subject, including two relatively recent works written by Eckhart Tolle that I would particularly recommend.[22,23] While meditation has been widely used for stress reduction in the West, it has traditionally been a part of spiritual practice, mainly in monasteries. As such, it is part of a way of life.

The true goals of Eastern spiritual practices are twofold—to enable experience of higher consciousness while at the same time

THE EAGLE'S WAY

weakening identification with the separate ego. Islam allows only abstract images in its temples and calls the faithful to prayer five times a day, which may help loosen their attachment to the busy mind.

Older Eastern religions take it further. Hinduism, Jainism, and Buddhism all have terms we translate as 'enlightenment.' The Hindus use the word *moksha*, which means liberation from desire and other-worldly passions. They see human life as a series of lives in different bodies until this final phase of enlightenment. The Mandukyu Upanishad sees *moksha* as a state of freedom from the ignorance that causes suffering. The idea is not to know God as a different being but to know one's real self and its essential nature, which is the Self of all.[24] The origins of Jainism are uncertain, but its organized form dates from sixth to ninth century BC. The highest form of knowledge the soul can attain is called *Kevala Jnana*, meaning "absolute or perfect."

Attained by spiritual discipline and ascetic practice, it alludes to *"infinite knowledge of self and non-self."*[25]

To the Buddhist, *bodhi* means awakening and understanding—an insight into the workings of the mind, which keeps humans imprisoned in craving, suffering, and rebirth. Bodhi brings a deep revelation into the meaning and purpose of all things and a fundamental alteration of consciousness whereby everything is perceived in unity.[26]

Research in 2004 lent some credence to the long-standing belief that spiritual discipline can increase the scope and quality of awareness. Neuroscientists at the University of Wisconsin compared the brain function of eight of the Dalai Lama's most experienced practitioners with a control group of student volunteers with only a week of training. The monks had considerably more gamma wave activity before they started to meditate, and that gap increased greatly once in meditation.[27] Christian scriptures have also hinted at this pathway of letting go of the ego as illustrated here:

> *For whosoever will save his life shall lose it:*
> *And whosoever will lose his life for my sake*
> *shall find it.*[28]
> *Except a grain of wheat fall into the ground*

and die, it abideth alone:
But if it die, it bringeth forth much fruit.
He that loveth his life shall lose it:
He that hateth his life in this world shall keep
it unto life eternal.[29]

Nevertheless it is essential for one to establish an ego before one tries to let it go. Much of psychotherapy is helping to develop a coherent, integrated ego, a very worthy and important function. Sanyasis, who leave behind the worldly life of India in pursuit of the spiritual quest, are usually over fifty years of age, a time when most of one's ego pursuits have been accomplished.

Benefits of the Inner Pathway

Where humans differ from the other life forms on earth is in their capacity to awaken to this great truth—to be conscious of it. Once people awaken to the reality of their true nature as consciousness, they open their awareness to a realm of immortality, love, power, and healing. The words *love, eternal life,* and *consciousness* are descriptive of a spiritual reality beyond intellectual understanding.

While these terms cannot be intellectually grasped, they can be experienced. An analogy can be made with electricity. In 2012, we still do not have a clear understanding of the nature of electricity. Yet we can still plug into it and benefit from its power. In a similar way, it is possible to 'plug into' deeper states of consciousness, thereby experiencing love, peace, and a sense of harmony with life.

One of the benefits of connecting with higher consciousness is healing, which is why this book gives considerable focus to this aspect of life. Our true essence, our 'I' entity, is one with all of life. It is hard to find a better definition of wholeness than this—and health is another word for wholeness.

Becoming aware of consciousness as one's true identity is called *awakening* or *being born again of the spirit.* However it is only a first step. This step is *recognition* of one's being as one with the collective, universal consciousness. Only after training and spiritual discipline

THE EAGLE'S WAY

does this recognition become habitual and real—a term described as *self-realisation*. With realisation comes *manifestation*. Self-realised beings manifest this state of being by having a sense of peace and charisma about them.

This journey inward is known by many names. The 'mystic path,' the 'road to enlightenment,' and the 'Tao' (translates as "the Way") are some of them. Throughout history, there have been people who followed this path and achieved self-realisation. They have been known by many names: sages, magi, seers, prophets, wise men, gurus, masters, wizards, and avatars among them. Stories of miracles surround these people—not just the biblical ones like Jesus and Moses but Krishna, Buddha, and many others too.

The miracles Jesus manifested are well known. Less so the miracles wrought by his followers. Paul spoke of spiritual gifts, two of which were healing the sick and working miracles.[30] If miracles and healing were as widespread as suggested in the Acts of the Apostles, it is little wonder Christianity spread like a grass fire in the first century AD.[31]

History of the Ancient Wisdom

The capacity to perform 'miracles' ensured self-realised beings an enthusiastic following. However, their followers rarely had the same understanding as these wise people. So the records of a master's words are often incomplete or distorted by the perceptions of the biographer. Later translations and rewritings can amplify these distortions.

A further complication has been that most of this ancient wisdom has been deliberately concealed from the mass of humanity. It has been considered important to keep this knowledge secret as knowledge brings power. For such power to fall into the hands of people with insufficient wisdom to safely use it was considered dangerous. Such people could use these powers for selfish ends—a practice called 'black magic.'

Mystery schools and secret societies were one way of restricting the ancient wisdom. Esoteric branches of mainstream religions were another. *Esoteric* is defined as "understood by only a small number of people"[32] and came from the Greek word meaning 'inner or internal.'

It has come into use to describe the inner focus on religious experience in contrast to the exoteric focus on religious faith. Secret codes, sacred languages, hieroglyphs, alchemical symbols, allegories, parables, and myths were other means used to transmit knowledge publicly in a way that would only be recognized by those ready to awaken.[33]

Esoteric Knowledge Comes Out of the Closet

Not until the late nineteenth century did esoteric literature start to appear in the public domain, and even then it was only a trickle. While the ideas behind quantum physics and the collective unconscious were articulated in the early part of the twentieth century, the 1960s saw them enter the popular consciousness. The hippie culture seemed to create an environment receptive to such ideas. A new interest in mysticism surfaced.

Perhaps the drugs, especially hallucinogens, were a factor. The hippies were having mystical experiences on magic mushrooms, peyote, and LSD. However, these substances could also cause frightening and dangerous trips. Meditation offered a safer route to one's inner world—a pathway remaining under one's own control.

In 1977, George Lucas started the *Star Wars* trilogy of movies that became the highest grossing movies of the era. The movies featured Jedi knights whose mission was to learn to trust *the Force*. The Force was an energy existing everywhere in the cosmos. As a concept, it was not unlike the quantum field and the collective unconscious. Darth Vader had trained as a Jedi knight but had lost his way and was misusing the Force for selfish purposes. The master, Yoda, sitting silently and calmly, utilized the Force appropriately, working miracles by so doing. The *Star Wars* films gave a demonstration of mystic principles. They showed why esoteric information had been kept secret. Yoda was a practitioner of 'white magic.' Darth Vader's misuse was 'black magic.'

Yet fears of misuse do not seem to have put any dent in the dissemination of esoteric books and writings. When I started reading mystical literature in 1980, there were only two bookstores in Melbourne where I could buy them. By 1990, there were twenty

THE EAGLE'S WAY

stores specializing in these types of books. Nowadays, virtually every conventional bookshop carries a section devoted to esoteric knowledge under headings of New Age, psychology, or health. In 2020, there is an abundance of websites to supplement the books.

Back on the bookshelves and the Internet is astrology, both Western and Chinese. Astrology started its resurgence around the 1960s. Despite its lack of scientific rationale, people are still finding meaning in it.

CHAPTER 10

Embracing Illness

Whether practitioners use conventional or alternative methods of treatment, faith, hope, and love remain the mainstays of the healing art. To the holistic practitioner, however, love is not only the most important aspect of the art of medicine. It is also the most important ingredient in the science of medicine. Love is the glue that connects individuals to themselves and to each other. It is a connection that is so important in maintaining health. As one philosopher put it, "*A healing occurs when one knows one's connection to the entire fabric of the universe.*"[1]

Making Love, Not War

"Make love, not war" was the catchphrase of the Flower Power Movement of the sixties. As a group, the hippies advocated peace and free love. They rejected the conventional values of the times, especially sexual suppression and the Vietnam War. Yet in another way, this catchphrase encapsulates the spirit of alternative medicine, changes that also emerged in the era of 'flower power.'

Making war against disease is all about fighting. Fighting disease or avoiding it corresponds to fight or flight, the instinctive reaction to fear. Both these strategies treat the disease as though it were separate from the patient. The purpose then is to put a greater distance

THE EAGLE'S WAY

between it and the patient—preferably by removing it altogether. Disease is seen as an evil that has invaded or befallen the body—an alien force that must be eradicated to re-establish the body's integrity.

While fear seeks separation, love seeks unity. Love embraces disease as an integral part of the individual. People who take an accepting attitude to disease utilize their illnesses as messages from their souls, letting them know that something is amiss. These messages can provide an indication as to what is actually missing in their lives. I have called this attitude of accepting illness and disease rather than fighting or avoiding it *the eagle's way* as it represents a way of exploring problems and rising above them. Rather than making war against the messenger, the eagle's way is to embrace it. Listening to the message and then working with the message to re-establish inner harmony and ease can allow the disease to go into remission. An example would be conditions like tennis elbow or inflammation of the tendons around the wrist. The obvious message is to give those parts of the body a rest because they are being overused. Influenza may be giving the body a message it needs a brief but total rest. Other messages may be much more subtle but in theory *when the purpose of a disease is no longer relevant, neither is the disease.*

The message may just be that it is time to leave the planet, especially in the elderly. Nevertheless healing can still occur at emotional, mental, and spiritual levels, when physical recovery is not in the soul's interest. Healing at these levels can bring a deeper level of inner peace, and integrity. To carry the analogy of a storm, eagles would not treat a storm as an enemy. Being caught in a storm would be an indication they were flying too low. The storm acts as a pointer to a higher and better way.

Love and embracing

It is not that there is anything wrong with fighting disease. Despite the limitations already mentioned, fighting disease is effective. Nevertheless, love as a force is superior to fear. Love can overcome fear. How much more energy do people have for doing things they love to do compared with doing things they are forced to do? To induce someone to do something for which they have no passion is likely to require some sort of carrot in front of them or a whip behind. But no inducement is needed to encourage people to do what they enjoy doing.

I have heard it said that the most powerful instinct in human life is self-preservation. Yet so many times people ignore this instinct and risk their lives to rescue others in emergencies. Not infrequently, people have drowned trying to save complete strangers. In such circumstances, the first instinct of the hero has not been self-preservation or concern for his or her own safety. It has been compassion for others. Love has proved stronger than fear.

Love is a broad term and as such, it is a difficult word to use in the medical sense. The ancient Greeks used four different words to describe love between people. *Eros* was romantic love with sexual attraction; *philia* was friendship of the loyal, dispassionate type; *storge* was the love between parents and children and *agape* was unconditional love, the highest form.

Agape comes closest and is like the English word compassion. I have used the word *embrace* as it means "to include or contain, to accept or support willingly."[2] This latter definition encapsulates the holistic approach and differentiates it from the purely conventional medical approach. While mainstream medicine fights disease, holistic medicine embraces it.

Embracing Life—The Holistic Perspective

Over the next three chapters, holistic medicine will be explored not only with respect to disease but also in relation to potential causes of disease. The role of relationships and other issues relating to health care will be elaborated.

The differences between the mainstream and holistic approaches will become more obvious as we consider those aspects of life related to health. These are listed under the following headings:

1.   Embracing pain
2.   Embracing disease

3. Embracing expanded consciousness
4. Embracing subtle energies
5. Embracing the power of intention
6. Embracing the power of imagination
7. Embracing emotions
8. Embracing beliefs
9. Embracing the shadow
10. Embracing intuition
11. Embracing spirituality
12. Embracing non-pathological psychological symptoms
    - Sadness and depression
    - Psychosis
    - Hallucinations
    - Synchronicities
13. Embracing people's experiences as truth
14. Embracing relationships
15. Embracing enemies
16. Embracing all systems of healing
17. Embracing healing unto death
18. Embracing all that is

Embracing Pain

The relief of pain and suffering remains a vital role in health care. Sometimes physicians choose to inflict short-term pain in order to avoid or relieve more serious suffering. Nevertheless, the principle remains. The importance of helping relieve a patient's distress is central to medicine. Hippocrates described a physician's role as this: "*To cure sometimes, to help always, to harm never.*"[3]

The work of Ainslie Meares

For many years, I assumed pain could only be relieved by using pain-killers or by curing the cause of the pain. Then, in 1981, I attended a talk given by Dr. Ainslie Meares, a Melbourne psychiatrist with a special interest in hypnosis. He believed pain and suffering were

DR. PETER L. JOHNSTON

two separate problems that were usually but not invariably present at the same time. To him, pain was a message from the body telling the patient something was wrong. Suffering, on the other hand, was defined more in terms of how the patient interpreted the pain.

When I enjoy a spicy curry accompanied with red wine, I frequently experience pain in the chest and upper abdomen. However, knowing the pain to be heartburn and knowing I can relieve it with antacids, my level of suffering is minimal. On the other hand, chest pain in a patient who has had no previous history of heartburn, no spicy food, and a family history of early death from heart attack could be a very different matter. Fear of death might engender considerable anxiety. This would in turn increase the intensity of the pain, which would in turn increase the suffering, creating a vicious cycle of pain and suffering.

Ainslie Meares surprised me by suggesting that pain in its pure state did not hurt. He had learned this from a very old Nepalese yogi who lived in serenity, meditating for sixteen hours per day. If the yogi stood on a nail, he would feel the pain, but it would not hurt. Dr. Meares also noticed how relaxed he felt in the presence of this teacher.

Meares then started sitting in uncomfortable postures and noticed how the discomfort disappeared after a few minutes of meditation. He further experimented by having dental procedures without local anaesthetic. On one occasion, he felt a lot of crunching and pulling as the dentist cut away bone to extract an impacted molar, but it did not hurt him.[4]

He led our group of family practitioners into a meditation in which we attached sharp paper clips to the backs of our hands. He told us to go into the pain, not push it away. The paper clip initially caused us pain, but as we embraced the pain and relaxed into it, we no longer felt any discomfort.

Ainslie Meares spent the last decade of his life teaching cancer patients to meditate. He helped many of them to reduce their pain. By doing so, they gained some sense of control over the severity of their suffering. In some cases, their meditation altered the course of their disease. A few of his patients achieved complete remission from their diseases.

THE EAGLE'S WAY

Losing the fight against chronic pain

Chronic pain is on the increase in Australia and the USA. Fighting it with pain-relieving opioids has been disappointing in that they rarely give complete relief, even with increasingly strong narcotics like Fentanyl.

Worse news is that the rates of addiction and deaths from overdoses of these drugs is rising steeply. Here in Australia, GPs are being urged not only to stop prescribing these drugs but to try to wean all their patients off them.

How to embrace pain

Gallstones and kidney stones cause no pain when they remain in the gallbladder and kidney. But once they stray into their collecting tubes, they obstruct the flow of bile or urine, resulting in severe pain known as biliary colic and renal colic. The muscular walls of these tubes contract forcefully to try to push the stones out of the way and re-establish flow.

So these severe pains are letting us know something is blocking the free flow of essential body fluids. We doctors give our patients intramuscular or intravenous opioids to reduce the pain but we know we have to relieve the obstruction to cure the problem.

Using the same analogy, e-motions are energies in motion. As long as we feel our negative emotions and then let them go, they pass out of our body.

However, when we hang onto resentment towards somebody because we are not going to let them get away with it, whatever 'it' may be, we are not allowing that energy to pass through. It sits there in our bodies like an energetic obstruction to the flow of life energies.

So, rather than fight pain with medications, the eagle's way is to embrace the pain, feel it and ask the pain what it is trying to tell you. Rest assured there is a deeper wisdom within you that knows exactly what is happening.

The answer may come in a memory of an event, a thought, a picture of somebody – and sometimes a sinking feeling that has

155

Personal experiences

In the seventies, when I was practicing midwifery, I was impressed with the ability of some women to go through labour without having narcotic analgesia. These women had practiced yoga or attended natural childbirth classes during their pregnancies.

In the eighties, many of my patients who had cancer attended a meditation group. Most of these patients gained better control of their pain as a result. Almost without exception, they gained a greater sense of peace that enabled them to face death more calmly.

When patients go into altered states of consciousness during a process called *breathwork*, they frequently encounter pains in various areas of the body. When they do, we encourage the patients to imagine breathing into the site of the pain. Often this takes them into experiences where they visualise themselves being injured in the area of the pain. We then encourage them to stay with the painful experience, regardless of how traumatic it may seem. Once the episode has reached completion, the pain subsides. Usually, the patients feel a sense of release and relief on completing these experiences. Dr. Stanislav Grof, the founder of *holotropic breathwork*, has seen situations where chronic pain has completely resolved once the episode, complete with its painful emotions, has been relived.[5]

While, on one hand, patients are encouraged to embrace their pain at times as part of the healing process, they are also advised to use analgesics when required. Adequate pain relief is very important. Chronic pain not only impairs one's quality of life but also saps morale and faith—and hence, it interferes with healing. So while courage is a virtue, stoicism can be a handicap. Embracing pain and fighting it are both appropriate at different times. As will be stressed many times in this book, there are no absolute rights and wrongs. There is a place for all. Balance is the key.

Embracing Disease

A scientific approach to health starts with the assumption of a cause for all disease. However, the cause of chronic disease remains unclear in most circumstances. Certainly, the role of microbes, allergens, and carcinogens in disease has been well documented. These represent the common external causes of illness.

The role of the patient's immune system in disease has also become clearer. The arrival of the AIDS epidemic has led to much research into the immune system. As well as the AIDS virus, malignant growths involving the immune system can also severely undermine the body's defence system. In such situations, normally friendly microbes can bring about serious, life-threatening diseases.

While not as spectacular in its effects, stress has been shown to have a negative effect on the immune system. *Psychoneuroimmunology* is a scientific field studying the connections between the mind, the nervous system, and the immune system. While the biochemical understanding is still in progress, this research has shown that one's mental and emotional states affect the immune system. Happiness, humour, calmness, and clarity are associated with good immune function,[6] while fear, anger, and depression are not.[7]

While the medical profession acknowledges stress as a factor in the cause of disease, an understanding of the different types of stress is still in the early stages of research. Epidemiological studies have linked heart disease with type-A personalities—impatient, ambitious, hard-driving, competitive people who are usually male. Research also suggests cancer patients may have a tendency to suppress their emotions, but these findings are tentative.[8]

Medical metaphysics

My simplified translation of the meaning of metaphysics is 'beyond physics.' *Medical metaphysics* is a term used to describe the non-physical (beyond physical) origins of disease. Basic to metaphysics is an understanding that disease in the physical body may derive from disharmony in the more subtle energy realms of mind, emotions, and will. In other words, an inner problem may manifest in physical illness and the form of that illness may provide a clue to the inner origin.

My earliest recollections of the connection between illness and the soul came from art. In Donnizetti's opera, *Lucia de Lammamor,* Lucia goes insane after she is pressured to marry against her will. Boris Pasternak's hero, Doctor Zhivago, dying of ischaemic heart disease at forty-two, uses these words:

> *Your health is bound to be affected if, day after day, you say the opposite of what you feel, if you grovel before what you dislike and rejoice at what brings you nothing but misfortune. Your nervous system isn't a fiction. It's a part of your physical body and your soul exists in space and is inside you, like the teeth in your head. You can't keep violating it with impunity.*[9]

The first exposure I had to medical metaphysics came in 1981 when I read some of the works of Dr. Edward Bach (1886-1936).[10] He saw disease as the result of inner conflict between the goals of the soul and those of the personality. Then in 1984, Louise Hay published a book listing approximately 350 diseases and symptoms together with their metaphysical causes.[11] In recent years, there have been a number of books ascribing metaphysical causes to a range of common diseases. Medical practitioners with skills in intuitive diagnosis have written some of these books.[12]

It needs to be said that inner conflicts do not always lead to illness and illness is not always the result of inner conflicts. However if inner problems are longstanding and unrecognized they may do so. While scientific validation is lacking, there is at least the recognition that emotional stress leads to a lowering in efficiency of the body's defence system, which in turn opens the body to viruses, bacteria, tumours and other diseases.

While I found Louise Hay's book helpful in making diagnoses, it became clear to me that each person is unique. The conflicts at the root of disease reflect that individuality, so no two patients have identical metaphysical causes for their illness. Over recent years, I have put less focus on trying to diagnose the metaphysical causes of disease and have aimed at helping patients to discover the causes for themselves.

However, there is one ancient healing system that provides not only a useful map for medical metaphysics but also an energetic bridge from the metaphysical to the physical. While it lacks scientific validation it has served the yogis well.

The chakra-nadi system of ancient India

The Ayervedic system of medicine in India has a universal energy, a life force they call *prana*. In the human body, the prana enters primarily through the breath, something shared universally. Prana is distributed throughout the body via channels called *nadis*, which are invisible to the naked eye. There are hundreds of these small ducts of energy interlinking with centres of energy called *chakras*, a term derived from the Sanskrit word meaning 'wheel.' These centres are vortices of energy that spin, and to the clairvoyant, they do indeed resemble a wheel. Although there are many chakras in the body and opinions differ about their relative importance, there are seven major chakras located centrally from the base of the spine up to the crown of the head about which there seems to be general agreement.

On a visit to Western Samoa in 1985, I developed back pain and visited a *fofo,* an indigenous healer. Without asking me about my health, she instinctively put her hands on the sore spot and eased the pain. Later, back at Aggie Grey's hotel, I met an American lady, the wife of a Samoan chieftain, who was doing research for her doctorate on the healers of Samoa. She showed me her drawings of the focal centres of their healing tradition. These focal points were at similar sites to the seven chakra positions of the yogic system. My assumption was that they must have imported their healing traditions from the East. But she was quite sure the Polynesian healers had found these centres independently through their own clairvoyant faculties.

Caroline Myss, a well-known writer and medical intuitive, realized after many years of doing intuitive readings for Dr. Sheally that she, too, had been focusing on these seven centres in the body without prior knowledge of the chakra system.[12] In concert with intuitive diagnosticians, hands-on healers, and dowsers, I have found a consistency in these energy centres that has convinced me of their existence. However, at this time, pranic energy cannot be accurately measured, and therefore, it falls outside the scientific paradigm.

These major chakras are like centres for the processing of energy—in both directions. Energies from the soul, the mind, and the emotions send their subtle vibrations to the chakras, which translate the energy to a frequency that can be tolerated by the body. From there, the energy goes to two twin channels called the *ida* and *pingala*, which travel on either side of the spinal cord and which translate and transmit the energies to the spinal cord and brain. In addition to the nervous system, each chakra is related to an endocrine gland so that hormonal flow to the physical body is also controlled through the chakra-nadi system. In the other direction, the messages from the body are all fed back to the chakras. The feedback from the body comes not only from the five senses but also from the balancing organ, muscular tone, and all the other organs that pass messages around the body to keep it as healthy as possible.

The base chakra

Otherwise known as the 'root chakra' (or *muladhara* in Sanskrit), this vortex of energy sits at the base of the spine just below the coccyx bone in the perineum. Its task is to coordinate everything related to security. I think of it as *security headquarters*. It is all about feeling safe on the earth—having food, clothing, shelter, structure, boundaries, warmth, and nurturing. For most of us, this is provided by parents, with additional help from family, friends, neighbours, and the community. Security involves a sense of belonging to the family, the tribe, and the environment in which we grow. It is this sense of finding our place that provides the 'base' of our existence. Children do not like playing on their own. They prefer to play under their mother's feet. The modern family room owes its popularity to this reality.

Insecurity activates the adrenal gland, the endocrine gland producing adrenaline and cortisone. These are the hormones that deal with the flight or fight response to fear and the ones that impel our bodies into these responses.

A positive archetype for this chakra is the *earth mother*. When people have this archetype operating, they feed and nourish themselves and provide their own nurturing. The negative archetype is the *victim*. When the victim is operating, people see themselves as being at the mercy of others and therefore dependent on the actions of others for their own security.

The base chakra is associated with the body's defence system. Severe dysfunctions can lead to immune deficiency diseases, including AIDS and chronic fatigue syndrome. It is also associated with the structural aspects of the body in keeping with its role in giving life a structure. Hence, the bony skeleton and disorders thereof are associated.

The sacral chakra

The Sanskrit name for this chakra is *Svadhisthana*, but it is often referred to as the 'sex chakra.' It operates at a level about five centimetres below the umbilicus. The key words to describe the scope of this energy vortex are "sensation, relationship, money, and sex." I refer to it as the *pleasure headquarters*.

The sacral chakra is associated with one-on-one relationships with partners, children, friends, colleagues, customers, and rivals. It is the centre for procreation and recreation. The extent to which people allow themselves pleasure dictates the amount of energy flowing through this chakra. Money is frequently associated with this chakra because it provides the means for much of life's pleasures. While money may be spent on essential, security, base-chakra energies of survival, the pleasure principle comes into play because people usually buy food, clothing, and shelter according to their tastes and desire for pleasure.

This chakra expands with pleasure and a sense of abundance and gratitude for life. It contracts with pain, poverty, and the denial of pleasure.

A positive archetype for this chakra is the *emperor/empress*. Money is not a problem for monarchs. They believe they are deserving of the good life. The polar opposite is the *martyr* archetype. Those with the *martyr* archetype deprive themselves of the pleasures of life.

The endocrine glands connected to the sacral chakra are the ovaries and testes. This chakra covers the activity of all the genital organs as well as the bladder and lower back. Dysfunction in this chakra can manifest as diseases of the prostate, bladder, uterus, ovaries, and fallopian tubes. Lower back pain is a common problem, often reflecting too much work or financial worries. These reflect the challenges of this chakra, which are about finding a happy balance between the pleasures of money, food, drink, relationships, and recreation and the work and discipline required to provide them.

The solar plexus chakra

The Sanskrit term is *Manipura*, and obviously, it acts at the level of the solar plexus, which is just below the sternum. To clairvoyants, its colour is yellow, the colour of the sun, which presumably is where the solar plexus derived its name. Its key words radiate who we are, namely "ego, self-esteem, identity, self-worth, integrity, gut instinct, and personal power." I think of this centre as the *headquarters for power and identity*. Whereas the lower two centres are related to relationships with the tribe and other individuals, this centre is all about the relationship with oneself. This centre becomes active when the ego develops in childhood, but it becomes the dominant chakra during the teenage years when it becomes important to establish an identity of one's own. Personal power forms from developing a sense of integrity in what one stands for and being able to hold to that sense of integrity through challenges and resistance. This enables people to grow in strength and character.

A positive archetype for this chakra is the *warrior*. With an empowered but not inflated ego, the warrior has the strength and determination to achieve his or her purpose. He/she is ready to fight the good fight for what he/she believes in. On the other hand, the less uplifting archetypes are the *people-pleaser* and *servant*. People dominated by these archetypes give their power away to others by

THE EAGLE'S WAY

seeking confirmation or approval from outside themselves, thereby allowing others to define their position or role in the world.

People's identities are usually centred on their roles, marital statuses, skills, genders, nationalities, and achievements. Or they may be centred around a group activity or a football team they follow. The highest thought that can flow through the solar plexus chakra is the one that comes down from the divine level, namely the truth that we are one with 'All that Is.' When this truth is known deeply, there is no longer a need to prove one's self. People know they are worthy just because they exist. They can love themselves unconditionally.

When there is a lack of personal power, the corresponding low self-esteem may result in a tendency to control or seek control by manipulative methods. There is a tendency to be extra-sensitive to criticism and a tendency to procrastination. On the other hand, if there is too much ego-based energy flowing through the chakra, there can be arrogance, the hunger for power, and the exploitation of others.

The endocrine gland here is the pancreas. The chakra processes energy to and from the liver, gall bladder, stomach, and small bowel, as well as the pancreas. Diseases like diabetes, gallstones, duodenal ulcers, cirrhosis of the liver, and food allergies are all conditions that will correlate with changed energy patterns in this chakra.

The heart chakra

The heart chakra (or *anahata*) is located in the centre of the chest. The key words to describe this centre are love, joy, peace, unity, brotherhood, and compassion—in short, the qualities that stem from an attitude of unconditional love. The heart chakra could be called the *headquarters for unconditional love*. Here, the relationships may involve the tribe, individuals, or one's self, but they take place at a higher level. Unlike the lower three chakras, where most of the energy is coming from the physical plane, the energy here is flowing from the higher spiritual energies into the physical.

The positive archetype is represented by the *lover*, which in archetypal terms means more than just the person 'in love.' The form of love implied here was called *agape* in ancient Greece to differenti-

163

ate it from romantic and sexual love, which they called *eros*. Agape describes a wider love that embraces not only one's partner and children but also humanity in total. This form of love is unconditional and inclusive of all, bringing respect for all creatures, compassion for human suffering, and a sense of awe at the perfection of the universe. When this archetype is operating, it brings a level of inner joy and peace that surpasses the pleasures of the lower three chakras. People transmit from the highest realms of the spirit. Love is given freely with joy, and it returns in like manner. People feel a sense of warmth, safety, and comfort when they are in the presence of the lover, precisely the sort of atmosphere in which growth and healing can take place.

By way of comparison, the *bigot* would describe a love that is conditional. For the bigot, love needs to be earned. Bigots have been conditioned to believe that certain people are untrustworthy, that some tribes are inferior, and that others are dangerous. Their love is quite exclusive and may exclude members of their own family if they feel such members have transgressed the boundaries of acceptable behaviour. Bigots are nevertheless capable of love, but the scope of their love is limited by their belief systems and expectations. If someone falls outside the bigot's definition of who or what is loveable, love is withheld and replaced by fear and sometimes hostility. We think of bigots as being prejudiced. The word *prejudice* comes from 'pre-judging,' namely applying judgement to people before even meeting them. They are judged to be unworthy because they work for the tax department or wear nose-rings. Lovers, by contrast, embrace them all just because they exist, knowing intuitively that anything or anybody in existence has a role in the life of the whole.

Thoughts that flow through this centre involve one's attitudes about love, about one's own worthiness to give and receive love, as well as the worthiness of others. The emotions emanating from a balanced chakra are love, joy, and compassion, while blockages may lead to hatred, fear, sadness, depression, and resentment.

The heart chakra connects with the thymus gland, an endocrine organ that usually has its maximum size and impact at birth and in early infancy. It forms an important component of the developing immune system but shrinks with age. It may not be just coincidental that the thymus shrinks as we develop the belief systems that limit our capacity to give out the unconditional love with which we start earthly life.

The organs associated with the heart chakra are the lungs, breasts, circulatory system, and the heart itself. Chronic problems with the energy flow through this chakra may manifest physically in these organs with diseases like hypertension, coronary artery disease, asthma, emphysema, and breast cancer.

The throat chakra

The throat chakra or *vishuddha* emanates from the level of the neck and throat. The key words for this energy are creativity, will, communication, honesty, and integrity. My term for this is the *headquarters for communication and intent.*

What lifts man above the animal kingdom is the capacity for thought, reflection, and speech. Thoughts and beliefs find their outlet in speech, and the extent to which these honestly reflect individuality is the measure of a healthy flow of energy through this chakra. As well as thoughts and reflections, people also express emotion through speech. When words reflect genuine emotions, there is a congruity that gives strength to the ideas being put forward. However, if people are mouthing words to conform to social expectations but do not sincerely believe in them, their body language will not match the words and will produce an incongruity conveying to others a feeling of insincerity.

The *authentic communicator* is an archetype describing the positive aspects of the art of communication, encouraging people to live from a sense of personal integrity. They can say no when they need to, and they 'walk their talk' so that there is no gap between what they say and what they do.

As a negative archetype, the closest character I can find is the *shamed individual.* This, sadly, is not an uncommon trait. Children who have grown up surrounded by personal criticism can form an attitude that there is some fundamental flaw in their make-up. As a result, they lack the confidence to believe in themselves, to back their

DR. PETER L. JOHNSTON

own judgement, or to communicate about themselves. They feel that nobody will be interested in their ideas, so they remain silent. If they do speak, they are likely to look for safety by saying what they feel others want to hear rather than what they might truly feel.

The throat chakra connects with the thyroid gland and parathyroid glands in the neck. Its energies influence the other organs in the area, namely the jaw, oesophagus, mouth, ears, trachea (windpipe), larynx (voice box), and the neck itself. Disorders of this area include sore throats, laryngitis, thyroid disorders, mouth ulcers, and ear infections.

The brow chakra

While the Sanskrit name for the brow chakra is *ajna*, it is best known as the *third eye* because when this chakra is fully opened and activated, the subtle organs of perception, especially clairvoyance, begin to function. However, it is also known as the control centre as it is the centre for the mind.

The brow transmits the energy that carries the capacity for clear thinking, intelligence, knowledge, imagination, intuition, discernment, and wisdom. These are the key words associated with the energy passing from the higher realms into the physical. However, this chakra also provides the means by which the subtle energies can be received into the conscious mind via the extrasensory perceptions of clairvoyance, clairaudience, and clairsentience. I think of this as the *mental headquarter*. As with all my chakra titles, it is an oversimplification, but I find it helps my understanding.

The thoughts that flow through the *ajna* can be harmonious or conflicting. When people are at peace with themselves, their thoughts flow quietly, almost imperceptibly, and provide a more complete and holistic view of the issues in focus. Both the left and right hemispheres of the brain are brought into play. When people are unhappy, stressed, and self-critical, their minds are busy and divided. It can be a struggle to find satisfactory answers to problems. At these times, the answers people find frequently contain the seeds of the next problem.

THE EAGLE'S WAY

Emotions of all types flow through the *ajna*, but it is here where the choice is made whether to allow emotional energy to be expressed, delayed, or suppressed. This is the control centre as far as allowing thoughts and emotions to flow into this three-dimensional realm. Once they are admitted, thoughts and emotions then flow through the throat chakra for their expression.

The positive archetype is the *sage* or *crone*, a person of wisdom who helps and guides others with a sense of adventure and trust. Sages have an interest in the meaning of life and go wherever their quest leads them. The *intellectual*, by way of comparison, may attain a vast amount of knowledge but limits it to rational, analytic, left-brain information. By excluding the spiritual and emotional aspects of life, intellectual academic knowledge lacks the holistic perspective and becomes a bit dry.

As befits the control chakra, it connects with the pituitary gland, also known as the 'master gland.' This endocrine gland secretes hormones that control the functions of the other endocrine glands. It also secretes the *growth hormone* that controls the overall growth of the body. It is an interesting reflection that growth in the mental, emotional, and spiritual aspects of life depends on the choices people make at this chakra level. Uplifting and adventurous thoughts, beliefs, and feelings enhance growth while negative, self-critical, separating, or fearful thoughts hold one back.

The main organs associated with this chakra are the eyes and the brainstem. Disorders include inflammations of the various layers of the eye, glaucoma, cataracts, blindness, headaches, and migraines.

The crown chakra

The crown chakra (*sahasraha*) transmits the highest energies of spirit. In the Eastern esoteric traditions, a beam of white light or spiritual energy called the *antakharana* enters the body through the crown and meets the physical energy from the earth entering through the base chakra.

The key life issue with this chakra is unity—the realisation of one's unity with all that is. Beyond the ego is this connection and

167

oneness with all of life. At a lesser but still vitally important level is the need for meaning—a life purpose that can be a rudder for one's choices and experiences. I refer to it as the *spiritual headquarters*. The key words associated with a balanced crown chakra are grace, ease, beauty, serenity, and oneness.

The thoughts that emanate from the crown chakra are holistic, global, and compassionate in their attitude toward self and others. Such thoughts take in a bigger picture of a conflict and provide the inspiration for a win-win outcome. The emotion associated with this chakra is bliss, which is defined as perfect happiness and joy.

The Western archetype for this would be what Maslow referred to as the '*self-actualised person.*' In the East, they would call such a person an *awakened one.* Such individuals have actually realised who they are and live and act from this sense of self. They have ceased to identify themselves purely as their egos. This brings release from the fears characteristic of human life and brings an aura of peace that stays with them, and it also brings healing to others who come into their presence.

This is in contrast with *unawakened people* who perceive they are totally separate from everybody else, who think they must work hard and compete with others to get what they want. They know only the ego, which they think is their true self. So they can find themselves in a dog-eat-dog world.

The crown chakra connects with the pineal gland, the function of which we are still discovering. We do know that its hormones affect our sensitivity to light and sleep cycles. *Melatonin,* which is one of its hormones, is currently being used commercially as a sedative and a drug to reduce the deleterious effects of jet lag.

The parts of the body associated with this chakra are the cerebral cortex and upper parts of the skull. Diseases like insomnia, epilepsy, Alzheimer's disease, and the neurological manifestations of alcoholism have been attributed to blockages in the crown chakra.

THE EAGLE'S WAY

Importance of Taking Responsibility but Not Blame

When disease is seen purely as a curse inflicted upon people at random, illness becomes just a matter of bad luck. There is no power in this. People afflicted by chronic disease become powerless victims. Looking for some meaning can change this. Taking responsibility for one's illness brings power. The word *responsibility* is derived from the words 'ability to respond.' If one takes responsibility for the situation, one can start to change it. Unfortunately, our culture tends to associate responsibility with blame. Stephen Levine uses the term *responsible to* rather than *responsible for*. I like this approach as it puts the focus on the response to the disease in the present rather than the feeling of being responsible for creating a disease in the first place.[13]

Lest this be seen as a punitive theory that puts further blame and guilt upon someone already suffering, it is important to make four points.

The first is to stress that disease is not a punishment or a moral judgement. The purpose of life is growth. Following what one likes to do is the best way to achieve this. Nevertheless, no two people are the same. What produces happiness for one person might give total boredom to another. There can be no hard and fast rules for individual happiness other than following one's heart. For each person, what brings joy at a young age may be totally unsatisfying at a later period in life. As people grow, tastes change. Whether it concerns relationships, work, or hobbies, the heart knows the way and needs to lead. When a person's heartfelt desire is blocked by another person or by the individual's own fear of change, inner conflict ensues. If this conflict remains unresolved, chronic disease could result. Even so, the disease would represent an attempt on the part of the soul to direct the personality toward a state of harmony. Failing to detect or act upon an early warning is not a crime. Failure is an inevitable accompaniment to growth. Without a few falls, a child cannot learn to walk.

The second point is to emphasise the "no blame" clause. While inner conflict may arise because of clashing beliefs, repressed emotions, or mixed intentions, such conflicts are not intentionally produced. More often than not, the conflict is unconscious. In fact, if it were conscious, the individual may well have resolved it. Beliefs can be absorbed from parents and siblings or pushed by zealous teachers before a child has the capacity to assess such beliefs. How can blame be attributed to childhood conditioning, hereditary characteristics, or confusion when a child has no say in these? Why should people be blamed for inability to express emotions like grief and anger when their culture discourages expression of those emotions?

Thirdly, if disease is a message from the soul, then the soul has directed the body to manifest disease for a purpose. While the purpose may be to bring attention to a conflict between the soul and the personality, this is not always the case. There comes a time when people have completed their missions on earth. Because their missions are defined in soul terms rather than by earthly achievements, individuals may not realise their work is done. But the soul knows, and disease may be the way in which the soul allows the individual to leave earth at the appropriate time.

Fourthly, the inner causes of disease are part of the vast mystery of life. Spiritually enlightened masters might die painfully while tyrants die peacefully in bed at ninety. At the level of soul (psyche), there is no separation. All souls are part of the collective unconscious. Perhaps a soul may elect to manifest disease for the benefit of others. The way in which a close friend of mine handled dying from motor neurone disease was inspiring to those around him.

A case history

An unforgettable patient was Karen, a fourteen-year-old girl. Karen was very intelligent, and she had a special talent for music. She developed a malignant sarcoma. During her illness, I explored her life and family thoroughly and could find no inner conflict. She radiated vitality and love of life. Being in her presence was an absolute joy. I used to look forward to seeing her, even though it was heart-wrenching to see her disease progressing. She did not give way to self-pity, fear, or depression. She expressed some of her deepest feelings in poetry. She was truly an inspiration to all who met her. I am sure her disease was not a wake-up call for her. Perhaps it was a message of love and courage to inspire others?

So while disease may be a mystery or a way to terminate human life, it might also be a call to change and grow. I believe it's well worth exploring.

CHAPTER 11

Embracing The Non-Physical Causes Of Illness

When illness or disease is reflecting a deeper inner conflict there are a number of areas where conflict can occur. Among them are the following:

- Repressed emotions
- Dysfunctional thoughts or beliefs
- Denial
- Conflicting intentions
- Shame and guilt
- Ignoring intuition
- Chronic resentment with unresolved hostilities
- Toxic subtle energies

In this chapter, we will explore some of these non-physical contributors to illness, highlighting the differences between the holistic and mainstream approaches.

Embracing Expanded Consciousness

Mainstream medicine views consciousness as a state of being awake and aware of one's surroundings. When people are asleep, concussed, or comatose, they are described as unconscious. People may be in coma and needing assistance to breathe, but if they have a heartbeat and brain waves on an EEG, they are considered alive. A flat line on a patient's ECG combined with absence of brain-wave activity on their EEG indicates that life has ended.

Yet people who are dreaming—and even those who are flat-lining after a cardiac arrest—can be fully aware of their surroundings. The difference is that their surroundings are not necessarily those around their body. Their consciousness is not in their body—it is elsewhere. If people spend an average of eight hours sleeping, their consciousness is only in their bodies for two thirds of their earthly lives.

To the holistic practitioner, consciousness is life. Other descriptions of consciousness are soul, psyche, and spirit. In sleep, consciousness takes leave of the body temporarily. In death, consciousness leaves the body permanently. The body then starts a process of decomposition. While scientific materialism sees death as the end of consciousness, spiritual traditions, including the great religions, see consciousness as continuing in other dimensions of reality.

Proof of the existence of life after death seems beyond the reach of scientists at this time. A common response I hear is this: "Nobody has returned from the dead to confirm this theory."

Yet most cultures have some concept of life after death. The four gospels all describe the reappearance of Jesus after his crucifixion, suggesting at least one man made a comeback.

Eastern religions, such as Hinduism, Jainism, and Sikhism, believe individual souls reincarnate in different bodies. In Tibetan Buddhism, the Dalai Lama and high-ranking lamas are recognized in their childhood because they choose the prayer wheels and beads belonging to their previous lives as monks or lamas.

It is likely the early Christians believed in reincarnation also, as Jesus is quoted as saying that John the Baptist was the prophet Elijah, who lived eight hundred years earlier.[1] People asked the master if a man's sin had caused him to be born blind. While Jesus answered in the negative, the question implies a life before birth.[2]

Dr. Helen Wambach, a psychotherapist, described hundreds of past-life regressions in her work with hypnosis, including many who described their current life purpose in relationship to events in past incarnations.[3] Dr. Brian Weiss was a traditional psychotherapist until one of his patients went into a past life under hypnosis. The patient also brought forward remarkably accurate information about the practitioner's own deceased son. From that moment on, Dr. Weiss used past-life therapy with his patients and found these psychic journeys were able to heal many of their emotional and physical wounds.[4]

In altered states of consciousness induced by breathwork, I have seen patients go into visual experiences in which they relive part of a life set in historical times. In most of these settings, the patients experience death. Yet afterward, they feel better for the experience. I have also undergone similar experiences myself under the supervision of transpersonal counsellors and breathworkers.

Dr. Ian Stevenson spent nearly forty years investigating over two thousand children. Without the use of hypnosis, breathwork, or any other mind-expanding technique, he interviewed children who spontaneously recalled past lives. He recorded his findings in ten books. Also available is a summary of his work by Tom Schroder.[5]

Embracing Subtle Energies

The word 'subtle' derives from the Latin word *subtilis,* meaning 'finely woven,' and it is defined as "delicate, faint, or not immediately obvious." In health care, it refers to those less visible energies surrounding and interpenetrating the body. Alternative practitioners refer to it as the *aura*, and it can be seen by the naked eye as a shimmering effect around a person's body when viewed against a plain-coloured background.

These subtle energies can also be detected with kinesiology, dowsing implements, bio-energetic instruments, and Kirlian photography. At this time, however, these energies cannot be accurately measured or quantified. The energies are also in a constant state of flux, making it difficult to use them as an aid to conventional diagnosis. Hence, conventional medicine does not embrace these subtle energies.

Although conventional medical practitioners are using acupuncture widely, there is a reluctance to accept the traditional explanation for its effectiveness. In 2005, *TIME Magazine's* "Year in Medicine" feature opened with this sentence: "*There is growing scientific evidence that acupuncture, a pillar of Chinese Medicine, can relieve many kinds of pain, but there's no clear agreement about how it works.*"

The Chinese themselves have no such misgivings about the mechanism of acupuncture. They have always maintained their belief in the existence of channels called *meridians,* carrying *chi,* a subtle energy. Meridians can be demonstrated using kinesiology, while Kirlian photography shows enhanced energy over acupuncture points. However, as neither chi nor meridians can be measured accurately, Western scientists are looking to endorphins and other biochemical explanations to explain why acupuncture works.

The chakra-nadi system runs into the same problem as these energies also cannot be accurately measured.

Embracing the Power of Intention

The 'will to live' is a very important indicator for success in conventional medicine. Without the will to live, a patient might not even consult a health practitioner. When people are forced to seek treatment, medical interventions are not often successful unless the patient develops a more positive attitude. This is a major problem in treating young women with anorexia nervosa.

Conventional medical approaches to health care do indeed embrace the power of intention. The holistic approach differs only in the degree to which it embraces this power.

The secular world uses the expression "the power of the mind" to explain some of the amazing events in life, especially triumph over adversity. Yet in most cases, the power of the mind is more the power of intention applied with trust and persistence.

Holistic medicine embraces the power of intention but is not secular. It embraces the concept of spirit or consciousness. The individual mind is not separate from the collective mind—the ultimate, creative intelligence known in religious traditions as God. With a connection of that magnitude, the mind is potentially very powerful indeed—capable of healing any illness.

Secondly, holistic medicine embraces metaphysics. From the metaphysical perspective, disease can arise from inner conflict—in particular, conflict between the goals of the soul and those of the personality. One of the major causes of inner conflict is frustration of one's life purpose. Hence, it is important to explore the values, goals, and intentions the patient holds dear. It is valuable to bring them into consciousness and see where they are being blocked, ignored, or lacking in clarity. Developing strategies to achieve those goals are basic to healing as well as being fundamental to personal happiness.

A case history

A sad but instructive story of the power of intention to affect disease was that of Madeleine. Aged forty-eight, Madeleine was dying of cancer when we first met. She had come to our local hospital because she did not want to die in a public hospital. Her breast cancer had spread to her liver and bones. She was bedridden because of a cancer-induced fracture of the hip. She had constant pain and intractable nausea and vomiting. I expected she would live no more than one to two weeks and arranged for her to have a private room.

In concert with a supportive director of nursing, we set out to make Madeleine's last days comfortable. In addition to analgesic and anti-nausea medication, we allowed her to use her own complementary remedies and practitioners. Given responsibility for her own health, she thrived on it. Within days of starting her own regime, her nausea and vomiting settled. She managed her pain by just rubbing flower essence cream into the skin over her fracture. Her whole demeanour lifted. One month later, she was walking on crutches, and her abnormal liver function tests had improved significantly. With the help of a Reiki practitioner, she became aware of how she had allowed herself to be the proverbial doormat to her husband and children. She began to assert herself and felt better for doing so.

Over the next six weeks, her progress seemed to plateau. Being a religious person, she asked her Reiki channel a question. "When is God going to make me better?" The answer she received was this: "When you yourself decide to get better." Instantly, she seemed to recognise her death wish. While in hospital, she could control her life and was happy, but she did not want to go home. She saw her marriage as dead. Her sons were independent and preoccupied with their own lives. Despite the efforts of friends, she could not see a future life or career for herself. When she realised she was choosing to die, her pain and nausea returned. Over the remaining few days of her life, even a hundred milligrams of morphine per day did not fully control her pain.

Embracing Imagination

The clearer one's intention, the more power it has to manifest. Recent research into neuroplasticity is showing how the brain creates neural pathways according to the intensity and frequency with which we focus on any subject of interest.[6] Hence, the more we focus on disease and illness, the more we reinforce those pathways. And it doesn't matter if that focus is antagonistic toward the illness. It still keeps the focus on the disease and strengthens the very thing we don't want.

The focus needs to be on health, not disease. However, if illness is the current reality, then wellness needs to be kept in the forefront of the mind and may require discipline, affirmations, and visualization to create the desired outcome, complete with neural pathways to maintain it.

Affirmations are positive statements embodying the desired outcome. They need to be in the present tense and be believable. The concept of 'autosuggestion' had its origins in the early twentieth century when Emile van Coue found that imagination was a stronger force than the will in achieving goals. His most famous affirmation was "*every day in every way I am feeling better and better.*" 'Coueism' became popular in Western Europe and United States after World War I and has had something of a revival in the 1980s. Constantly repeating positive goals with intensity and faith makes sense in view of the recent findings on neuroplasticity.

A really strong way of building positive pathways is to visualise the desired goal. The clearer the image of what we want, the easier it

DR. PETER L. JOHNSTON

is for the body to produce it. It's not unlike an architect's drawings. They act like a template for the ultimate physical result.

A Case History

The first time Justin came into my consulting room, he announced he had cancer. Only forty-eight, aggressive prostate cancer had already spread to his pelvis, skull, and ribs. He was taking hormones, but it was not checking the relentless progress of his malignancy. He joined a cancer support group that encouraged silent meditation in the Ainslie Meares method. However, Justin's style of meditation was more active. He could see his bones, and he'd clean them each time.

After he had been doing this for a few months, his wife rang me up in distress, telling me that Justin was depressed because he thought that he was getting worse. She told me he would be asking me to organize for a bone scan to assess his progress and asked me to not to tell him if the news was grim. She felt he wouldn't cope with it. I explained as best I could my need to be honest with Justin, who did indeed arrive soon after and took with him a request for a total-body bone scan.

He returned to the surgery two days later, looking anxious. His anxiety was contagious. I felt butterflies in my stomach as I went to search for the imaging report. To my surprise, it read, "No bony metastases noted." I immediately rang the radiologist to check if he had reported on the correct patient. When he confirmed it, I suggested he check Justin's previous bone scan. He came back to the phone and said, "I see what you mean. It is interesting. Must be spontaneous remission." I have never seen depression lift so suddenly as when I showed Justin the results of his bone scan. Later in our discussion, I asked him what had led to his low state of morale prior to the scan. He replied, "When I meditated, I couldn't see my bones anymore." As soon as he said it, he laughed, realizing he'd completed the job of cleaning up his bones.

Embracing Emotions

Emotions are important in psychiatry. However, psychiatrists mainly see people when their emotions are excessive—when they are suffering from depression, chronic anxiety, mania, or panic attacks. In the mainstream, the psychiatric approach is to try to reduce or relieve the patient's symptoms. This may involve using anti-depressive or tranquillising medication.

Emotions are described as positive when they connect with being happy. Love, joy, enthusiasm, elation, acceptance, ecstasy, and empathy are examples. Less happy states of being, such as fear, panic, anger, disgust, boredom, shame, and grief, are classed as negative. As a general guide, positive emotions connect people with their environment and are love-based. Negative emotions give people the feeling they would prefer to be separate from the people, things, or events producing the emotions.

For the holistic practitioner, all emotions are important, whether they are (a) normal or excessive, (b) suppressed or expressed, (c) recognised or unrecognised, and (d) positive or negative.

Emotions are the most accurate measure of how people truly feel about the relationships, events, and situations of their lives. As such, it is important to embrace all of them. Accepting all emotional states as being valid for each person at that particular time is part of the healing process. Therapy may well involve attempting to transform negative emotions, but first, they must be identified and accepted. As mentioned earlier, it is the judgement of emotions as being wrong that causes many of the problems. When people have been conditioned to believe anger is bad and crying is unmanly, it can be difficult for them to express their feelings.

While medications may be used at times, holistic practitioners usually do not use them without first exploring the emotions and trying to help the patient view their distress from a different perspective. The goal of healing is to embrace emotions, not to fight or suppress them. The value of embracing emotions will be explored in more detail in Chapter 12.

Embracing Beliefs

When emotions can be freely expressed, beliefs underpinning negative or suppressed emotions can be seen more clearly. Children have been told, "Do what you're told and don't answer back." "Big boys don't cry." "Children should be seen and not heard." "Money is the root of all evil." Such statements from authority figures may become dysfunctional beliefs. Those beliefs can still wield remarkable power in the lives of those children when they become adults.

Other beliefs may never have been stated but may have been inferred: "One should be competent at everything in order to be of value." "It is important to be popular . . . or look as though one is." "One's actions require the approval of others."

More frequent and more crippling are beliefs about one's self. Thoughts of being inadequate, unlovable, insignificant, unattractive, powerless, and even useless may arise from painful past experiences or criticisms from important authority figures and peers. These are powerfully negative beliefs that generate shame. Shame automatically causes inner conflict. The soul or higher consciousness knows the inherent beauty of the individual. Shame is a denial of this. So the personality is in conflict with the soul.

Yet these beliefs will not tumble out in normal conversation. In some people, they may only be semiconscious or even unconscious. People may only become aware of their presence when they are able to freely express their emotions and realise the negative beliefs underneath. It is unpleasant to find negative self-beliefs lurking in one's mind, but it is better to know they are there. Ignorance is not bliss. Negative beliefs create negative outcomes regardless of whether the beliefs are conscious or not. At least awareness allows the beliefs to be examined and changed.

Hence, the importance of finding them and embracing them, taking them out, looking at them, and bringing them into the light. Like all dark thoughts, they lose most of their power when brought to the light. They can be seen for the garbage they are. Most are false conclusions based on scant evidence. When harsh, destructive criticism is examined, it can often be seen to have arisen from the critic's

THE EAGLE'S WAY

own pain or frustration. Having the courage to embrace one's dark beliefs pays dividends. Knowledge replaces ignorance and denial, bringing new power to the individual.

Embracing the Shadow

The *shadow* was a term used by Carl Jung to define those aspects of our nature we would rather not see. Jung saw the collective unconscious as containing a vast reservoir of *archetypes—patterns* of thinking, feeling, and acting. Examples of these archetypes are *earth mother, perfectionist, businessman, rebel, warrior, sage, hero, doting father, nomad,* and *artist.* The people who demonstrate these archetypal patterns in their lives tend to show definite attributes regardless of their nationality or culture.[7]

A child has the capacity to embrace any archetype, but the family and culture tend to accept and praise some archetypes while the group discourages others. For example, parents who desire peace and harmony in their homes may encourage the *peacemaker* and *giver* archetypes in their children while they may discourage the *warrior* and *taker* archetypes. If the children have the *people-pleaser* archetype, they will oblige their parents by becoming peace-loving, selfless children. Their selfish traits along with their warlike capacities become suppressed. These attributes, however, do not actually go away. They form part of the child's shadow. Children will continue to act selfishly, but covertly rather than overtly, as they will not want to appear selfish. Their warrior sides, while disowned, are also likely to erupt, given sufficient provocation, and that eruption might well be volatile when it breaks through the suppression. These disowned archetypes are projected outward onto others. So when these unselfish, peace-loving children meet others who seem selfish or aggressive, they will have an emotional response to them—either repulsion or attraction. They will tend to love them or loathe them instead of just accepting them.[8]

The same process of projection occurs at the national level. No doubt it is more comfortable to see evil in dictators, terrorists, and criminals. By directing attacks against them, leaders can see themselves as heroes fighting evil. The evil is projected away from them.

DR. PETER L. JOHNSTON

However, because humanity shares in the collective unconscious, we are all capable of reaching the depths of the worst criminals and the heights of the great saints. A cartoon I saw many years ago by Pogo put it succinctly. A Native-American forward scout, his hand shading his eyes, announced, "We have sighted the enemy." He then turned, and with a quizzical look on his face, he said, "And it's us!"

It is the judgement of archetypes as bad that causes them to be discouraged in the first place. In the Christian tradition, the "seven deadly sins" were seen as inherently evil. On the other hand, *patience* is not necessarily a virtue when someone needs urgent, life-saving resuscitation. Some degree of *sloth* is essential to balance a busy working life in order to prevent burnout, while relationship problems can be helped with a good dose of conjugal *lust*.

In general holistic approaches are not about defining absolute rights and wrongs. Aggression and even homicide can be justified in self-defence and praised in warfare. In holistic counselling, all archetypes are embraced, especially those disowned ones hiding in the shadow.

The Greek gods had flaws as well as virtues. Some were good examples of common archetypes. Hal Stone, who discovered a system for communicating with archetypes, was fond of saying this: "*It was acceptable for ancient Greeks to have their favourite gods, but it was essential for them to honour all the gods in the pantheon.*"[9]

Embracing Intuition

Intuition is defined as "the ability to understand something immediately without the need for conscious reasoning." I think of it as 'tuition from within'. While everybody has intuitive ability, some seem to have it in abundance. They usually have clairvoyant and clairaudient faculties in childhood. If they find someone who understands their gift and helps them develop it, they become adept at reading this 'language of the soul'.

Because science is based on conscious reasoning, it has an uneasy relationship with intuition. Scientists use terms such as hunches and "gut instinct," which are synonyms for intuition, but they do not

THE EAGLE'S WAY

always see these responses as reliable. Sometimes, when their hunches prove to be accurate, credit is given to rational thinking and their ability to detect subtle clues.

By contrast, holistic practitioners view intuition as a potentially accurate source of information. While rational thinking emanates from the conscious mind, intuition has at its disposal not only conscious data but all the vast resources of the unconscious. However I use the word potential because any extra-sensory perception (ESP) may be distorted by the attitudes of the individual receiving it.

In 1985, Dr. Norman Shealy, founder of the American Holistic Medical Association, met Caroline Myss. Caroline felt she had some capacity for picking up people's emotional and physical problems. When Dr. Shealy had a patient in his consulting room, he would ring Caroline, tell her the patient's name and birth date, and ask for her impressions. Most of her initial responses detailed the conflicts in a patient's life, but as Dr. Shealy pressed her to look at the physical, she began to intuitively enter each patient's body and speak as though she were the patient. Her accuracy was astounding. He requested her help with hundreds of patients over a period of eight years, and her physical diagnoses coincided with Dr. Shealy's in 93 per cent of cases. It was more accurate than his MRI scans. But in addition to the physical diagnosis, her readings included causal factors at the emotional, mental, and spiritual levels, so a patient had an opportunity to explore lifestyle therapeutic options.[10]

Since then, intuitive diagnosis has become a sub-specialty of its own. People who have developed their intuitive skills can detect energy changes in areas of the body where disorders exist. Gifted intuitives can tune in to the frequencies of this energy and read the message encoded in this energy, which can be helpful for clients seeking healing.

I have been referring patients to intuitive diagnosticians since 1997. I have found their contributions helpful for those patients prepared to consult with them. However, unlike technology, humans do have their off days, and scientific medicine needs reliability. Mainstream medicine has not embraced intuitive diagnosis as it is

DR. PETER L. JOHNSTON

considered too subjective. Hence, it is likely that intuitive diagnosis will remain complementary rather than enter the mainstream.

What intuitive diagnosis does demonstrate is the existence of inner knowledge of disease. The intuitive is reading information from energies within and around the patient. Obviously, this knowledge is available to the patient. Yet the patient may not be consciously aware of it. However, when the patient hears the information, there is usually a clear recognition of its truth. It may be information the patient has been reluctant to acknowledge. Patients may not be ready to see that their hearts are no longer in their jobs, roles, or relationships. They may not be ready to change to a healthier diet or lifestyle.

Because intuition is constantly trying to give important information, it makes sense to listen to its tuition. Some form of meditation practice is helpful in doing this. Herbert Benson performed scientific studies on devotees of Zen, yoga and transcendental meditation in the sixties and seventies.[11] These and subsequent studies showed enough health benefits for insurance companies to offer reduced premiums to people who meditated regularly. Although meditation and yoga are not mainstream therapies, they are accepted more readily as complementary approaches by the mainstream.

CHAPTER 12

Embracing The Whole

Embracing Spirituality

As previously mentioned, scientific medicine in the twentieth century has been secular in its approach. Mainstream psychiatry and psychology have taken a similar tack. With scientific progress, religion and spirituality have been viewed as belonging to a more primitive, unscientific era of superstition—a time when there was a need for greater reliance on prayer and magic.

Secular cosmology starts with the big bang theory. Out of the big bang came the galaxies, stars, and planets. Single-cell organisms emerged from the waters of planet Earth. From these primitive life forms, plants and animals evolved. Humans evolved from apes and went through some primitive forms before their brains developed the current shape of *Homo sapiens*. In this secular, scientific approach to creation, matter came first. Consciousness grew out of matter. The psyche or mind is located in the brain. Consciousness is the result of physiological processes within the brain—processes whose mechanisms are yet to be clarified.

Observations in transpersonal psychology have cast serious doubts on this theory. Many people have experienced consciousness outside their bodies, demonstrating the capacity for consciousness to operate independently of the brain. If consciousness is separate from

DR. PETER L. JOHNSTON

the body, it fits the definition of spirit or soul, both of which define consciousness in non-physical terms.

In reaffirming the non-material nature of consciousness, holistic medicine embraces spirituality to the point of restoring it to its central place in healing. Spirituality is concerned with finding meaning in one's life. Those whose philosophy of life has no place for survival after death can struggle when afflicted with life-threatening disease. On the other hand, an understanding of man's spiritual nature and his unity with the love that permeates the universe can bring peace of mind and harmony within.

Spiritual (transpersonal) experiences may occur in altered states of consciousness induced by hallucinogenic drugs or by therapies incorporating breathing techniques. They can also occur spontaneously in meditation or as "near-death experiences" in life-threatening illness. Regardless of their origins, such experiences can be transformational. A new understanding of life can emerge. A new direction can evolve, and existing diseases can regress after such an event in a person's life.[1] These spiritual experiences are like windows into a different reality.

Although they might only afford a brief glimpse at another realm, they can be an experience of awakening to a deeper truth. Teilhard de Chardin, the Jesuit palaeontologist and philosopher, put it beautifully when he inverted the situation with these words: "*We are not human beings having a spiritual experience. We are spiritual beings having a human experience.*"

Embracing Non-Pathological Symptoms

Mainstream psychiatry views certain symptoms as indicative of disease. Yet in some circumstances, these symptoms may be an indication of health. Like spiritual experiences, they can be diagnostic of a stage of transition on an aspirant's journey.

Depression

Major life changes often arise as a result of crisis. Whether it is bankruptcy, separation, or disillusionment with life as it is, a person finds the old ways no longer work. There is an inevitable stage of grief that goes with this situation. Frequently, a new door does not open until the old one is closed, so there is a void or vacuum in one's life. The old situation is depressing, but the new is not yet visible. This phase of life brings sadness for which counselling is helpful. However, for some, this sadness may plunge more deeply into depression and even suicide. In such situations, medication may be needed along with counselling.

There is another form of depression found in those who have entered a phase of 'spiritual awakening.' A Christian mystic described it as *'the dark night of the soul'.*[2] It can be a very dark state of mind, but it is the darkness that precedes the dawn. In centuries past, it was an event seen only in monasteries where the sufferer would have the support of his fellow monks or nuns. Nowadays, it can occur to anyone seeking spiritual enlightenment. Treating this form of depression with medication is interfering with a natural healing process that will ultimately lead to a deeper form of happiness and inner peace.

Psychosis

Spiritual awakening brings with it an expansion of consciousness and a weakening of limited beliefs. For some, this leads to brief periods of psychosis as the contents of the unconscious arise. Spiritual traditions have described this state as *divine madness*. Plato saw this state of "heaven-sent madness" as almost a prerequisite for successful priestesses and prophetesses in ancient Greece.[3]

In 1981, after months of absorption in esoteric reading, my powers of reasoning went into decline for a week, culminating in a day of psychotic behaviour. I was delusional and hallucinating. Fortunately, I found my way to a spiritual adviser before a psychiatrist found me. The following day, my mental state was stable again. A few years later, my wife, Nikki, came across a book written by Peter O'Connor, a psychologist who described a state of insanity provoked by awakening to a deeper spiritual reality. She gave it to me with a laugh, telling me I would really enjoy reading it. I did. It was certainly a relief![4]

Hallucinations

Clairvoyance and clairaudience, while viewed as extrasensory gifts in spiritual parlance, are seen as hallucinatory in medical and scientific circles. Unless someone invents a camera capable of imaging disembodied entities the whole arena of guides, ghosts, angels and the existence of life after death will remain controversial.

I have visited a few clairvoyants. Two of them accurately described deceased friends and relatives and passed on their greetings and messages. I have felt these were authentic as well as helpful and optimistic. Nevertheless without being able to see or hear these entities myself, intuition was my only guide. So I strongly recommend others when seeing clairvoyants to keep their own internal bullshit detectors operating.

Synchronicities

Classical science has no theoretical basis for understanding synchronicity. Conventional medicine and psychiatry, being grounded in classical science, see synchronicities as coincidences. As mentioned earlier, conventional medicine sees synchronicities as the results of chance.

When Jung first described synchronicity, he defined it as 'meaningful coincidence.' He saw synchronicity as a law that operated to draw people toward personal growth—to grow in consciousness and self-awareness. Synchronicities, far from being meaningless coincidences, were part of the cosmic order. They were life's way of leading individuals to find their own healing and life purpose.

Synchronicities are more common than many realize. Somebody I have not seen for a long time comes to mind. Within a short time, I run into him in the supermarket, or I receive a phone call from him. At other times I have been recommended to read a particular book by two or three people. I believe such coincidences are important to follow. I always buy a book if its title has come to my notice more than twice because I assume this is a message from the universal consciousness—a message to help me.

An anecdote

I was one of twenty-five attendees at a workshop on the subject of spiritual healing. We were divided into groups of three as a means of getting to know each other and sharing our reasons for coming to the workshop. Katherine, a young woman in her late thirties, had come in the hope of actually seeing spiritual healing occur rather than just hearing about it. Her preference was to find healing for her own arthritic pains. She spoke of the death of her partner five years before. The other member of our trio was a seventy-year-old lady who had also lost her husband five years earlier. Because my wife had also died five years earlier, it seemed an interesting coincidence.

What took Katherine by surprise was the extent to which the presenter, a psychiatrist, explored the emotional and personal aspects of life. I think she was expecting to see hands-on healing with no questions asked. She became agitated, eventually crying and asking the presenter to stop. She complained about not feeling safe within the group. The presenter listened to her with compassion. He suggested a bonding exercise for the group done to a musical background. Katherine agreed.

Within seconds of starting the exercise, Katherine was in full emotional catharsis. Unbeknownst to the presenter, he had chosen the very song Katherine and her partner had considered to be "their song." Her story came out in sobs. Her partner had committed suicide. She felt abandoned and betrayed. She had shut down emotionally and retreated to an isolated farm where she surrounded herself with animals. At least she could trust animals. She had lost faith in people.

As her tears flowed, the presenter asked if she would like any help from the group of if she would like a hug. She responded in the negative. She did not know anyone well enough for that. I thought the door of the conference room was completely closed, but just as the presenter asked that question, there was a squeaking noise as the

DR. PETER L. JOHNSTON

door slowly opened. A gray cat slinked through the door, walked up to Katherine, jumped into her lap, and snuggled in. It was an awesome moment for the whole group. Three synchronicities in one session were enough for me to know that the healing experience Katherine had sought was under way.

Embracing People's Experiences as Truth

There can be a tendency for physicians to question patients' experiences when they do not fit in with the physician's idea of what's possible.

Experience as a registrar in a maternity hospital gave me early exposure to this trait. Expectant mothers would arrive and say that their waters had broken. If, on examination, doctors observed either a tear in the sac or amniotic fluid in the vagina, the diagnosis would be confirmed. The patients would then be admitted to hospital, as ruptured membranes signified the likely onset of labour. If the doctor could see neither, patients were reassured their waters had not broken and were sent home. I heard more than one obstetrician telling his pregnant patient she must have mistaken urine for amniotic fluid.

Some years later, my wife, Nikki, experienced exactly the same routine, but it went a step further. After she was reassured she had passed urine and not amniotic fluid, she also told hospital staff she was having labour pains. They contacted a senior obstetrician. He put his hand on her abdomen and reassured the surrounding nurses that "this woman is not in labour." A few hours later, Nikki surprised the hospital staff by delivering a premature baby in difficult and dangerous circumstances.

The obstetrician was so certain of his own knowledge that he discounted the experience of the patient. Some of my own worst errors have come from not listening properly and jumping to a diagnosis without all the facts.

People who have transpersonal experiences can suffer the same fate. Because there is no room in the secular medical model for spiritual experiences, doctors view them as either being a product of the patient's imagination or as evidence of psychological instability.

My experience of fifty years in general practice tells me that patients' experiences are almost always genuine, even if I cannot explain them. With the exception of malingerers looking for a day off work and drug addicts looking for drugs, there is little point in not telling the truth. However, patients will withhold information, especially spiritual experiences, if they sense such information will fall outside the doctor's map of reality. The patient's intuition is no doubt protecting them from having their experiences ignored or invalidated. Many patients do not tell their doctors they are seeing alternative therapists or taking herbs if they know the doctor does not believe in such therapies.

As a practitioner of holistic medicine, I see it as important to trust in people's experience and embrace all they divulge to me. I feel very honoured when people trust me sufficiently to share their truth. Patients obviously did not trust me with their spiritual experiences during my first fifteen years of medical practice because no patient ever shared one with me. When I recall my cynicism of those years, I have to admire the wisdom of patients in not divulging their secrets. As a young graduate, I thought it was the doctor's job to have the answers, so I might well have spouted absolute nonsense in earlier years. Looking back, I am ever so grateful for what patients have shared with me. They have been my best teachers.

Embracing Relationships

In making out records for new patients, medical practitioners usually include a family history, mainly because some diseases are hereditary and other diseases have a tendency to recur within families. A patient's marital state is included, but the quality of the marital relationship is not of interest unless (a) the patient has come to see the doctor for advice about problems in the relationship, (b) the patient has a stress-related illness requiring exploration, or (c) the patient's illness is likely to have significant ramifications within his or her family.

Relationships, especially intimate ones, are of interest to holistic practitioners for all the above reasons as well as some additional ones.

Firstly, statistical studies have shown a lower incidence of illness generally in those who have good relationships with their spouses.[5]

Secondly, disease may be related to conflict or frustration with respect to one's purpose in life. Among the common goals in life are loving relationships with one's spouse and children.

Thirdly, Jung saw intimate relationships as playing a major role in spiritual growth. In those with no interest in personal growth or spirituality, relationship remains **the** main arena for growth—albeit an unconscious route. While couples may share common goals, hobbies, and traits in terms of archetypes, they often carry each other's shadow sides. For example, the intellectual and physically strong male may be attracted to the intuitive, emotional female. When they are in love, they are attracted to those qualities they have not fully developed in themselves. Their different approaches to life are something to celebrate. As a couple, they feel whole. When the magic wears off, the tendency is to criticise these qualities, comparing them unfavourably with their own. "Why can't she be logical and practical instead of being so emotional?" is the male's complaint while his partner is bemoaning his lack of sensitivity, understanding, and ability to give her thoughtful little surprises. This is where the real work of marriage starts. Over years of mutual love and tolerance, each partner absorbs a little of the other's traits and thereby becomes more whole as an individual.[6]

Harvill Hendrix also saw relationship as a subconscious growth process. Over years of marital therapy, he observed a tendency for individuals to seek out partners with similar attributes to one or other parent. He saw this as a subconscious desire to heal childhood wounds.

A young woman with an absent, workaholic father might be attracted to a man with similar traits. While logic would suggest she should be more interested in an attentive spouse, her soul desires attention and love from someone like her father. That way, she can heal her wounds as well as feel valued and loved.[7]

Fourthly, spouses can be a great source of help in assessing the underlying problems in patients. In some situations, they know the patients better than the patients know themselves.

Embracing Enemies

Enemies are a special variety of relationship. They are simply relationships one would rather not have at all. Nevertheless, they are still relationships, whether wanted or not. Energetically, enemies are connected. Emotions like hatred, resentment, and jealousy are energies. These negative energies are not just missiles on a search-and-destroy mission. They are boomerangs. The resentment directed toward another is resentment felt emotionally within the sender. Such negative emotions, if chronic, can not only cause negative moods like depression but also undermine the immune system and contribute to physical disease.

The sooner one can resolve a dispute with another, the better. Forgiveness is healing for the soul and body. While it may be necessary to feel the negative emotions involved in a traumatic event and even relive the event emotionally before one attempts forgiveness, completion of healing ultimately requires forgiveness.

Sorting out relationship conflicts is peripheral to conventional medicine because physical disease is not routinely seen as being connected to mental and emotional factors. Conversely, forgiveness is an important aspect of holistic health care.

Embracing All Health-Care Approaches

As a medical student in the sixties, the word 'quack' was freely used to describe any health practitioners using methods not approved by the medical profession. In those days, it referred mainly to chiropractors and osteopaths. Acupuncturists and naturopaths were a rare species then. The Medical Board of Australia still has a clause discouraging doctors from referring patients to those with unrecognised qualifications. However, with the majority of family practitioners using some form of complementary therapy themselves or sharing consulting suites with CAM therapists, this clause has become inactive.

Conventional medicine has no monopoly on this form of criticism. While I was studying naturopathy, I found some teachers to be quite critical of conventional medicine.

I believe all healing approaches have some merit, while no one system has the answer to all health problems. I look forward to a time when all health practitioners will view each other as colleagues. Nevertheless, alternative practitioners will not get recognition from the mainstream unless they have established educational institutions with appropriately qualified graduates. This process has gathered momentum over the last thirty years. Without research into their effectiveness, alternative therapies will also struggle for recognition from the mainstream. While double-blind trials could prove too expensive and difficult for most modalities, outcome studies could be sufficient for recognition. This would involve comparing the end result for patients under treatment with other patients who eschew that form of therapy.

Embracing Healing unto Death

As medical students trailing physicians on ward rounds in the sixties, we would stop at each bed and discuss the patient's illness, diagnosis, and treatment. However, dying patients were bypassed. Being beyond curing, they were the failures in the system.

While the dying may be beyond a physical cure, they are not beyond emotional or spiritual healing. If people resolve conflicts and emotional struggles, they are experiencing healing, even if their bodies are decaying. To overcome resentment and express forgiveness to another person is not only healing to the dying patient but also healing to the recipient.

Tibetan Buddhists emphasise compassion. Their monks place such importance on dying gracefully that they practise and rehearse for their last moments on earth. For them, the quality of their next incarnation depends on the degree of peace with which they leave this life.

Holistic practitioners may or may not believe in reincarnation, but they do believe in the continuity of consciousness. If the soul is immortal, then growth and healing are always possible. When critically ill people find inner peace, even physical healing has been known to occur.

Embracing All that Is

Embracing life and everything life brings is an ideal, but it's an ideal that can bring health. The capacity to accept the vicissitudes of life is a great gift. I really admire the phlegmatic personality who can remain grounded and unemotional in a personal crisis. These are not people suppressing their anxiety. They genuinely accept the fact that life will bring joy and sadness. Instead of spending time reacting and railing against their fate, they use their time and energy to formulate strategies to deal with the problem. It is as though they realise life is cosmos, not chaos. My intellectual search has led me to the same conclusion, but it seems to be stuck there in the mental realm, as volcanic eruptions can still form a part of my response to minor setbacks.

Failure, as a necessary step toward success, is something I understand intellectually. Acquiring skills, competence, and wisdom comes only through the experience of failure. Yet this intellectual knowing does not stop me from feeling anxious about failure.

Embracing "all that is" means accepting everything in life. It does not mean we have to like everything that happens, but it does imply accepting the reality of our lives. Not to do so is to live in denial. As the serenity prayer goes:

> "God, grant me the serenity to accept the
> things I cannot change,
> The courage to change the things I can And
> the wisdom to know the difference."

Accepting "all that is" does not mean accepting Third-World poverty as being desirable or something ordained by God. It may well be our purpose to help change it but it implies a trust that life does indeed have an order and a purpose, even if we cannot see it.

Larry Dossey, MD, wrote a book on the power of prayer called *Healing Words*. In addition to detailing the research findings validating the positive effect of prayer, he explored various methods of praying. He concluded that prayers of appreciation were likely to be more effective than entreaties for specific goals. He finishes his book

DR. PETER L. JOHNSTON

with this sentence: *"No longer will we pray incessantly for things, such as our health, but our prayers will be predominantly prayers of gratitude and thanksgiving—our proper response on realising that the world, at heart, is more glorious, benevolent and friendlier than we have recently supposed."*[8]

Pronoia is a word I am hearing lately. I have not seen it in a dictionary as yet, but I am sure it will soon be listed, as it is a word that has immense power if realised. It means the opposite of *paranoia*. People suffering from paranoia believe the world and the people in it are out to get them. They have suspicion and mistrust of people—delusions of persecution. Pronoia is the belief that *"all of creation is conspiring to shower us with blessings."*[9]

CHAPTER 13

Nourishing The Body

The focus of health care is ultimately the body. Over my lifetime, I have seen an increasing interest in healthy diet and lifestyle, but scientific findings on the best way to nurture our bodies have not always been conclusive.

Smoking

The deleterious effect of smoking, however, is one scientific finding that remains incontrovertible. Sir Austin Bradford-Hill pioneered the double-blind trial by testing streptomycin on fifty patients with tuberculosis in the early post-war period, when there was only enough streptomycin to treat a small number. Streptomycin proved to be effective, but all too soon, the tubercle bacillus developed resistance to it. From that time onward, it was never used alone to treat TB. It proved to be a very important finding, one that ultimately saved many lives.[1] Bradford-Hill, in concert with Richard Doll, turned his statistical skills to exploring lung cancer. Lung cancer had comprised 1 per cent of all cancers found at autopsy in 1878, but by the early twentieth century, it was contributing 10 to 15 per cent of all cancers. It represented 0.3 per cent of all autopsy findings in 1852 but 5.66 per cent in 1952.[2] Doll and his colleagues interviewed seven

DR. PETER L. JOHNSTON

hundred patients with lung cancer and became convinced that cigarette smoking was a major causal factor.

In 1950, they sent letters to every doctor in the United Kingdom, and forty thousand responded, detailing their smoking habits. Within five years, the connection was obvious. Smokers not only had a relatively higher incidence of lung cancer, but the incidence increased proportionately with the amount and duration of smoking. Smoking for thirty years was sixteen times more likely to produce lung cancer than smoking for fifteen years.

It was not a popular finding. Not till 1957 did the UK government hold a press conference, where the minister for health announced the government's acceptance of the report—in between puffs on his cigarette! It was 1964 before the surgeon general of the United States suggested that people stop smoking.[3] Personally, I took no notice of either of them!

The doctor's study continued for fifty years and helped implicate smoking in cancers of the lip, mouth, larynx, and oesophagus.[4] In 2002, warnings were extended with respect to smoking and cancer of the stomach,[5] kidney,[6] pancreas,[7] bladder,[8] and breast.[9,10] Long known to cause obstructive airways disease and lower birth-weight babies, smoking was also shown to increase the risk of cardiovascular disease, especially in people under forty years of age.[11,12]

Western Diet

As a schoolboy in the 1950s, we ate three meals a day at home and had half a pint of free milk at school during the morning break. Breakfast consisted of toast and cereal with milk. Lunch comprised sandwiches with cordial at junior school, but graduation to senior school brought with it a pie and a milkshake from the tuckshop.

We sat down to dinner as a family of seven in the evening. Meat, poultry, or fish was accompanied by thoroughly cooked vegetables. Finishing what was on our plates was compulsory. Dessert was standard, consisting usually of stewed or canned fruit accompanied by junket or custard (or on special occasions, ice cream).

When I started at medical school, I was expecting to learn all about nutrition. However, the six-year course was made up of three years in basic sciences followed by three years of clinical work in hospitals, and I cannot recall any lectures at all on nutrition. After graduation, four years of institutional food in hospitals and the army was just a continuation of the same.

With marriage came a change of chef and a new outlook on food. More through her own reading than any teaching in her nursing course, Nikki reserved dessert for dinner parties and special events only. Fruit was served raw and vegetables close to raw. Sausage meat, fried eggs on fried bread, and other fat-laden favourites of mine were removed from the menu, and roasts were cooked in water instead of lard.

Such changes seemed serendipitous because the typical Western diet, with its high content of animal fats, sugars, and dairy products and its low fibre component, was to come under more scrutiny in the seventies. Adding to the confusion was research suggesting that combining fruit with dairies and meat with veggies was an inefficient use of the body's enzymes.

Fibre

Dennis Burkitt, an English surgeon who went to Africa in the forties, noticed he was seeing little in the way of gastrointestinal diseases in the African people. Diverticulosis, bowel cancer, and even appendicitis were rarely sighted by comparison with the numbers he had become used to seeing in Britain. Yet when he studied the statistics on these diseases in the United States, they were just as common in African-born Americans as they were in the white population. Obviously, something in the native diet or lifestyle of Africans protected them from diseases of the intestines, and he thought it might be the amount of fibre in their diet.

At medical school, we were taught that diverticulosis was a common condition and that most westerners would show a few of these little pockets in the walls of their large bowel after the age of forty. When these pockets became inflamed, the treatment was a low-residue diet, namely a diet low in fibre in order to rest the bowel.

DR. PETER L. JOHNSTON

Burkitt's research brought a complete turnaround. Suddenly, the medical profession was recommending diets high in fibre, not only for patients with diverticulosis but for healthy people looking to stay healthy. Initially, bran and other heavy fibres were recommended, but later, it was found that better results came from eating raw vegetables, fruit skins, and softer fibre. However, the use of pesticides and the practice of polishing apples led to health-conscious people looking to organically grown fruit and vegetables.

Sugar

The connection between sugar and diabetes was well known. At school in the 1940s, we used to speak of "sugar diabetes" and feel great sympathy toward children who suffered from it, not just because they had to have injections every day but because they had to forgo ice cream, lollies, and chocolate.

A trip to Western Samoa in 1986 opened my eyes to the dangers of sugar and processed foods in general. A physician in Samoa informed us that diabetes was virtually unknown in the Pacific in the nineteenth century. Polynesians and Melanesians are solidly built constitutionally, but with the arrival of Western food, obesity increased—and with it diabetes. He made a special example of Nauru, a small island with a population around ten thousand. Once, the islanders had lived on tropical fruits and fish they caught in their outrigger canoes. The discovery of phosphates led to aggressive mining of the island. The result was a wealthy population but a lunar landscape with little remaining arable land. With plenty of imported processed food and less exercise, their weight increased to the extent that diabetes afflicted a quarter of the population, and it was affecting them at a younger age than the average westerner. Many of them were dying young. While he made an example of Nauru, he stressed that the problem belonged to all the islands of the Pacific and referred to diabetes and obesity as being caused by "the coca-colarization of the Pacific."

Not much has changed apparently. In 2019, 95% of Nauruans are considered overweight, 70% obese and 40% diabetic. Sadly, life expectancy for males has dropped to less than fifty. A recent survey

THE EAGLE'S WAY

measuring the extent of obesity in various countries has Nauru topping the list, followed by nine other Pacific Islands before Kuwait and USA filled eleventh and twelfth places.[13]

Fats

Apart from sugar, the other prominent component of the American and Australian diets has been saturated fats, which are fats derived from meat, dairy products, and eggs. In the fifties, Encel Keys found that Italians and Japanese who had little saturated fats in their diet had on average a much lower LDL cholesterol level, and raised LDL correlates to an increased rate of heart disease and strokes.[14] A later survey suggested heart disease was on the increase in the Western world, except in Italy, where it remained static. Conventional wisdom suggests that a diet high in red meat, saturated fat, sweets, white bread, and processed foods generally leads to a greater risk of heart disease. Conversely, a Mediterranean diet, high in fruit, vegetables, whole grains, fish, unsaturated fats from vegetable oils, especially olive oil, may lower the risk.

Red meat and the Western diet were also linked with bowel cancers. Sir Richard Doll, one of the world's most eminent cancer epidemiologists, published a review in 1981, suggesting food to be the cause of 35 per cent of all cancers.[15]

Reviewing the link between diet and disease

In recent years, several major studies have begun to reveal that fibre, while important, does not make any appreciable difference in colon cancer. Burkitt did put forward a second theory, but at the time, it was overlooked. Native Africans used the squatting position to defaecate, a posture that fully empties the colon and avoids waste entering the appendix. Research is now exploring the relationship between toileting posture and intestinal health.[16] The link between dietary fats and LDL cholesterol has remained controversial. Nathan Pritikin, on looking through records of autopsies on concentration camp detainees, found most had clean arteries. His diet was based on similar restrictions, and followers of it felt like they were grazing rather than eating. But without SS guards to police the diet, it was hard to stay with it. I have been recommending moderate reductions in sugar and fats to my patients for years but have to confess the reductions in LDL levels have been less than spectacular. Even cardiologists are now questioning whether diet really makes any difference to cholesterol levels in the blood. An analysis of published studies in 2010 found no clear link between people's intake of saturated fat and their risk of developing heart disease.[17]

Recent research has found that saturated fats found in coconut oil may actually be beneficial.[18] Studies have shown no significant difference in terms of weight control between taking skim, low-fat, and whole milk. In fact, taking the fat out of milk leaves too high a concentration of natural sugars.[19] Nuts, although high in fats and calories, can curb hunger and add valuable nutrients.

The link between food and cancer has never really been proven. Epidemiological studies showed that Argentineans with higher beef consumption have a lower rate of bowel cancer than people in the United States. Mormons, who eat meat, have lower rates of bowel cancer than Seventh Day Adventists, who are vegetarian.[20] Other studies have suggested sugar, refined carbohydrates, and fats, especially combinations thereof in the form of French fries, doughnuts, hot dogs, and processed meats, are carcinogenic. However, other studies have either contradicted or failed to support these findings.

Of interest has been the discovery of antioxidants, which are substances within the body keeping it from rusting, so to speak. Among the most valuable of our antioxidants are red wine, coffee, and chocolate, especially dark chocolate. All three have addictive qualities, and many healthy diets have recommended abstaining from them.

Food Intolerances

Having been told for years how essential cow's milk was for growth and metabolism, especially bones and teeth, it was surprising to hear it come under fire. While I had come across patients who were lactose intolerant, they seemed fairly uncommon. Yet most of my

THE EAGLE'S WAY

patients who visited naturopaths in the 1980s were being encouraged to remove dairy products, wheat, and yeast from their diets. At the time, I was sceptical of this advice, but in later years, when we used kinesiology and Vega machines to test for food intolerances, these three were among the most common foods to show up in patients with fatigue or chronic illness. Surprisingly, butter and yoghurt were frequently tolerated where milk and cheese were not.

Asians were nearly always found to be intolerant to dairies, probably because the dairy industry was not a part of their culture. Nevertheless, like Caucasian children, some of them had managed to get used to drinking milk by flavouring it. Once they stopped taking dairy products, they would crave them for a few weeks. After about six weeks, they would no longer want them or even like them. And their general energy—and often their behaviour—would improve. According to the National Osteoporosis Foundation of the United States, as many as 90 per cent of Asian Americans may be lactose intolerant. While they express concern about this, there is no evidence that osteoporosis is any more common among the Asian Americans than their Caucasian counterparts, suggesting they are finding sources of calcium other than dairy products.[21]

Gluten is a protein found mainly in wheat, oats, barley, and rye. People with coeliac disease cannot tolerate gluten. It produces atrophy of villi in the small intestine, which can be seen on endoscopy. Once diagnosed, a gluten-free diet is mandatory for life. Not so easily diagnosed but much more common is wheat intolerance, but this can be short-term or long-term. If somebody has been eating wheat for breakfast, lunch, morning tea, and sometimes dinner as I did for fifty years, it would be reasonable to suspect wheat intolerance as a possibility. If in addition there is a history of fatigue, bloating, flatulence, and a runny nose after eating bread or biscuits, the diagnosis is certain. Six weeks off wheat is a worthwhile trial of treatment after which wheat could be slowly reintroduced. While some people cannot tolerate wheat indefinitely, for most, it is just that the body wants a break from such a monotonous regime, and wheat can be resumed in moderation thereafter. In the United States, corn is a popular staple, and corn intolerance is found more frequently there.

203

DR. PETER L. JOHNSTON

It is important to differentiate intolerance from allergy. An allergy to a food like shellfish or peanuts is lifelong and life-threatening. Ingestion can cause instant distress from a rash to anaphylactic shock and cardiac arrest. Food intolerance is sometimes referred to as allergy addiction as that is the way it seems at times—a craving for a substance the body doesn't need. Intolerance to a food may arise from overuse, or it may just be an aversion to certain foods like Brussels sprouts. My aversion to the latter has lasted about sixty-five years, so it could be considered lifelong, whereas my intolerance to wheat is temporary but prone to recurrence when overindulged.

The inconsistency of food intolerances does not fit neatly into the conventional medical model. I first noticed this phenomenon in the early 70s. I saw migraine sufferers unable to tolerate red wine, cheese, or chocolate. Yet on an overseas holiday, they were able to drink generous quantities of French reds, blue cheese, and a few chocolates with no resultant headaches. I thought that something might be shifting for them, but back at home, despite good quality red wine and cheeses, their migraines returned.

With my own wheat and dairy intolerance, I noticed a similar response. When I felt happy and comfortable with my life, I could enjoy cappuccinos, hot cross buns, and even cheese melts with no ill effects; however, if my mood or energy was depleted, wheat or dairy products would produce uncomfortable symptoms, and I'd feel worse.

Traditional Chinese medicine with its focus on the life force or energy called chi goes closer to making sense of intermittent intolerances. I suspect food intolerances always deplete the body's energy levels.

Instead of the food providing energy, it uses up energy by forcing the body to protect itself from the consequences of the unwanted substance. But only when the body's energy levels are low does the body up the ante and let us know quite clearly to desist. For people suffering from fatigue states and chronic illness, eliminating any substances to which the person is intolerant or addicted is beneficial.

Elimination diets can be useful for healthy people too. It can enable one's intuition to guide food choices. The healthy pregnant woman who craves a pickled onion or a hamburger at 3:00 a.m. is

THE EAGLE'S WAY

responding to an instinctive need for a nutrient required by her or her baby. The person craving a Mars bar because he or she hasn't had one for an hour is responding to addiction. If food addictions can be eliminated from the diet, the body's natural urge can be trusted. We can then eat what we feel like and know it will be okay for us. Unlike drug addictions, most foods can be stopped cold turkey.

The Middle Path

While abstinence may be required to break addictions and intolerances, temperance is the virtue – moderation in all things. While sugar, fats and fast foods have not been proven to cause cancer, few would recommend using them as a staple. Humans have been consuming fruits, vegetables, grains, meat, fish and poultry for millennia, whereas processed foods are only recent additions to the human digestive tract. Practitioners of nutritional medicine recommend a 'rotating diet' to avoid developing food intolerances. When I eliminated wheat from my diet and replaced it with rye, I developed intolerance to rye within three weeks. It seems the body likes variety. On this basis, ingesting a variety of grains, fruits and vegetables makes sense.

The Adventist Health Study, a large survey done in 2014, showed that vegetarians, many of whom ate fish, had significantly lower incidence of bowel cancer than a control group. However, as a group, the vegetarians didn't smoke and rarely partook of alcohol. Hence making it difficult to draw conclusions on the role of diet. Nevertheless, in 2015, the World Health Organisation classified red meat as a possible carcinogen.

I've tried being vegetarian but have failed to persist with the discipline. So I admire those who stick with it. Some vegetarian patients don't like the taste of meat but most avoid it due to an aversion to hurting animals. And despite efforts to avoid cruelty, it still happens. Young calves are removed from their mothers within a few days, fed on milk or grains, often raised in group pens and slaughtered for veal at a young age. Baby veal may be only weeks old. Spring lambs are slaughtered at five to six months of age, while baby lambs may only live two months. The cruelty involved in battery hens is well known.

Red meat may not be good for human health and is clearly not great for animal health. But it's not good for global health either. A staggering 51% of global greenhouse gas emissions come from animal agriculture. The downside of vegetarianism is the difficulty providing the body with adequate protein, iron and vitamin B12. It takes considerable diligence to do so, especially when growing or menstruating.

Weight Reduction

Of course, the main reason for dieting is to lose weight. Obesity is a huge problem and becoming worse. More than 10 per cent of the world's population is obese, and rates have doubled since 1980. The biggest increases are in the richer nations, but most countries have seen rates rise.[22] Obesity tends to bring other health problems with it—diabetes, hypertension, cardiovascular disease, and osteoarthritis in hips and knees. Nevertheless, it is important to define obesity. Body mass index (or BMI) is a formula based on body weight divided by height. It has come to be the yardstick for adult weight classification. A BMI under twenty is considered to be underweight. A BMI between twenty and twenty-five is considered ideal. A BMI between twenty-five and thirty is generally judged to be overweight, while a BMI over thirty is labelled obese.

The importance of differentiating the latter two is highlighted by studies suggesting BMI is only predictive of longevity at statistical extremes. The very thin and the morbidly obese live shorter lives than the others do. Surveys have found that people who are overweight or mildly obese live at least as long as those in the ideal range and often longer.[23,24,25,26] Paradoxically, obese people with diabetes,[27] high blood pressure,[28] heart disease,[29,30,31] and kidney disease[32] live longer than thin people with these same conditions—and overweight senior citizens tend to live longer than their more slender peers.[33]

The obvious solution to obesity is to eat less and burn off more calories through exercise. There are many reduction diets available and new ones emerging all the time. Most have been built around diet and exercise. The medical profession has helped out with anorectic medication aimed at reducing appetite. For the morbidly obese, reducing the capacity of their stomachs by stapling has been a life-saving procedure in many cases.

Rick Kausman, a medical doctor specializing in the psychology of healthy weight management, observed a recurring pattern in dieting, one that he calls "the vicious cycle of a dieter."[34]

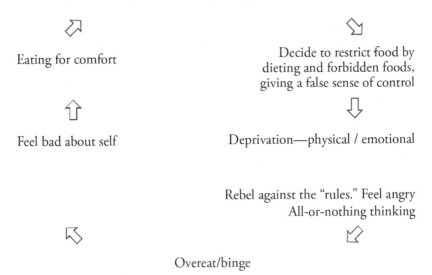

Recently, Rick's observations have received support from research in United States. Traci Mann of UCLA analysed thirty-one long-term studies on weight-reduction diets. She found that most people lost 5 to 10 per cent of their weight in the first six months but that weight loss was sustained only by a small minority. Most regained the weight within five years. In one study, 83 per cent regained more weight than they'd lost.[35] The longest randomised control dietary intervention study involved twenty thousand women. After eight years on a low-fat diet, reducing calorie intake by an average of 360 calories per day and increasing their activity, there was little change in weight from the starting point.[36]

DR. PETER L. JOHNSTON

A panel of experts at the National Institute of Health determined that one third to two thirds of dieters regain lost weight within twelve months and almost all have done so within five years. They summed up by saying: "There is little support for the notion that diets lead to lasting weight loss or health benefits."[37]

Worse, there have been a number of studies suggesting that going on and off diets does more harm than good.[38,39,40,41,42] Yo-yo dieting, rather than producing slim, healthy bodies, appears to be bringing about frustration, weight stigmatization, reduced self-esteem, and eating disorders.[43,44,45,46,47,48,49]

When Rick Kausmann looked at his vicious cycle and realized dieting was not the answer, it became clear the answer lay on the left side of the cycle—dealing with the guilt, bad feelings, and self-denigration. Two basic changes were required: desisting from judging foods and from judging one's self.

He declares food to be morally neutral. Words like junk food are to be avoided. Chocolate is not "bad." Nor apples "good." Chocolate can be life-saving to lost hikers, and recently, dark chocolate has had good press for its health-enhancing qualities. Rick prefers the terms "everyday food" to describe fruit, vegetables, and whole grains and "sometimes food" to describe party food and fast food.

He stresses the importance of eating slowly, recognizing when hunger has been sated, and stopping rather than finishing one's plate. Looking deeper for the causes of eating when not hungry is helpful too. Focusing on eating and enjoying the tastes of the food go with finding forms of exercise that are enjoyable. As eating is frequently a substitute for love and nurturing, he stresses the need for self-nurturing, not just in sport or exercise but in all aspects of life—reading, relationships, craft, crosswords, watching television, massage, etc.[50]

Health at Every Size (HAES) is a growing trans-disciplinary movement focusing on intuitive eating and pleasurable activity rather than dieting. They do not believe the healthy BMI range is maximally healthy for every individual. Their approach is for each person to eat in response to physical cues rather than emotional ones and to enjoy physical activity, thereby finding their personal ideal weights, which may well exceed BMI guidelines. They also define self-acceptance as "*affirmation and reinforcement of human beauty and worth irrespective of differences in size and shape.*"[51]

Nevertheless, the most vital ingredient is loving and accepting one's self, not just after successfully losing weight but before doing so. Self-acceptance allows one to maintain focus on the goal of reaching the desired appearance, whereas dissatisfaction keeps one focused on what one does not want. It helps to put away the scales and the full-length mirrors and keep reinforcing the desired body configuration.

It is a bit like a paradigm shift in weight management. The old paradigm resembled the following:

1. Optimal health and happiness require us to be slim.
2. We can all be slim if we try hard enough and think slim.
3. Overweight for an individual can be measured on a chart.
4. The cause is simple: gluttony, sloth, or a combination of both!
5. The solution is simply: reduce food intake and exercise more.

The new paradigm of weight management goes like this:

1. Health and vitality comes in all shapes and sizes.
2. We can lead happy and healthy lives without conforming to society's idea of an ideal shape.
3. Being above a comfortable weight is relative to the individual.
4. The causes of overweight are complex and multifactorial.
5. Solutions including setting realistic, individual sustainable goals.

Solutions need to be empowering to the individual and involve working on why specific issues have contributed.[52]

This new paradigm conforms to the eagle's way. Crash dieting is fighting the problem. Like birds fighting a storm, dieters get good short-term gains but get battered by the rebound phenomenon of bingeing. If they are not careful, they can also get buffeted by low blood sugar. Giving up on weight management allows one to rest in a comfort zone like birds opting for shelter from the storm, but no progress is made toward the goal.

DR. PETER L. JOHNSTON

The eagle's way accepts the presence of the black cloud of obesity but refuses to give it attention. Instead, the focus goes toward the goal—the desired body shape. In other words, the focus is on the solution, not the problem. While accepting the challenge of the dark cloud, there is trust in one's ability to rise above the challenge, establish long-term healthy eating habits, fun activities, and enjoyable exercise, and leave room to enjoy less wholesome treats every now and then without judgement.

CHAPTER 14

Love And Emotion In
The New Paradigm

The expression "God is love" was frequently mentioned by priests and teachers during my school years. I experienced some difficulty with this understanding of love as I was also informed this loving God was ready to park my soul in the everlasting fires of hell should I die in mortal sin. Given that the church interpreted all sexual transgressions, from fantasies to masturbation as mortal sins, hell seemed a hard place to avoid. Michelangelo's painting of the *Last Judgment* in the Sistine Chapel is an artistic masterpiece, but it's frightening nonetheless. God seemed a figure to fear rather than love.

The church viewed sex after marriage quite differently. Marital sex, being more about procreation than recreation, was deemed holy—wholly approved by God. So as a teenager, a quick mental wedding ceremony prior to entertaining sexual fantasies seemed to me a good way around this problem. However, my friends were not convinced such a tactical ploy would enable me to escape the last judgement. Fortunately, the last thirty years have brought new information—statistical data that casts the nature of the last judgement in a very different light.

DR. PETER L. JOHNSTON

Near-Death Experiences

Raymond Moody's book entitled *Life After Life,* first published in 1976, brought some lightness to this gloomy picture for me. Dr. Moody interviewed 150 people who had lost consciousness to the point where those around them thought they were dead.[1] Some twenty years later when Moody was interviewed, he had spoken to more than ten thousand people who had had near-death experiences (NDEs). He also asserted there were millions of NDE accounts described worldwide. From his own extensive experience, he repeatedly saw a definite progression of events in these NDEs.[2]

Stage 1: The out-of-body experience

At the time the doctors think the person has arrested or died, the patients say they drift up and out of their bodies. They can look down and see their own physical bodies lying there, surrounded by the medical personnel. While they watch the attempts to resuscitate them, the patients themselves have no pain, feel fine, and sometimes wonder what all the fuss is about. Some can recall the words and actions of their resuscitators.

Stage 2: The passage

As the near-death experience continues, people become aware of a passage of some sort. Most frequently, it is a tunnel, but some have described a bridge, a gateway, or a field through which they travel. Usually, they can see a light in the distance.

Stage 3: The light

Once through the passage, they enter the light—a light like no other light. As they enter, it envelops them with feelings of love, peace, and total acceptance. Professor Kenneth Ring, co-founder of the International Association for Near-Death Studies, describes this light as *the essence of what we ourselves are.*[3] According to thousands of reports, "In this light is all love, total acceptance, knowledge, complete perfection, warmth, and a beauty beyond our ability to imagine." He is describing something beyond the best concept we might have of ourselves.[4]

Dr. Elisabeth Kubler-Ross achieved fame for her pioneering work with the dying. Less well known has been her own work on NDEs. Over a period of thirty years, she and her team of counsellors interviewed more than twenty thousand people with NDEs. When Elisabeth experienced an NDE herself, she described it thus: *"I hastened towards the light and went smack into the centre of it. I literally melted into it, like falling into a water-bath of love. Suddenly, I became aware that this was Home, that we are part of this Light—that this is where we come from."*[5]

Stage 4: The life review

Many describe an incredibly loving personal presence that helps them review their lives. The review is about seeing what they have learned during their time on the Earth. It is always a loving process. Raymond Moody said he had never seen a single case of a person who had not been met with love and understanding in this process.[6] It remains a possibility for the actual experience of death to differ from the near-death experience. Nevertheless, unless Moody's large sample of NDEs were all saints, the last judgement would appear to be far more benign than the gospel translations have suggested.

Stage 5: The return

Few, if any, wish to leave the light. When they do, it is usually because they feel they have unfinished business here on the earth. When they do return, there is one lesson they have generally absorbed from the experience. Time after time, people who have had an NDE will say, "Learning how to love is the most important thing in life."[7]

DR. PETER L. JOHNSTON

Scientific Data

There have been scientific efforts to explain NDEs as hallucinatory experiences. While anoxia, metabolic dysfunctions, and toxicity from drugs can all produce hallucinations, there are some aspects of NDEs that seem to defy alternative scientific explanations.

During NDEs, people have travelled out of their bodies to the homes of relatives or friends. In an instant, they could be in the house of a loved one on the other side of the world. On returning, they have described scenes and actions that have later been verified as accurate. Dr. Moody told of a patient who arrested on the operating table. She was describing her NDE to a social worker soon after. While she had been floating above the hospital, she had noticed an old shoe dangling from a cable on the hospital roof. The social worker immediately went to the roof and retrieved the shoe from the exact place the patient had described.

Blind people, even those born blind, have been able to describe their experiences in visual terms—not only their inner experiences but also verifiable objects during their out-of-body experiences, things they would not have been able to see in their normal lives on the earth.[8] Hallucinations cannot explain these phenomena. Nor is it likely that pathological events would bring about the remarkable personal transformations that have occurred subsequent to NDEs.

A personal anecdote

I read Raymond Moody's book in 1981. It made quite an impact on me, but I remained somewhat sceptical. He was estimating that one in thirty people had NDEs, which suggested they were quite common events. Yet, despite talking to people for fifty hours per week for sixteen years, I had never heard anyone speak of having an NDE. Yet in the twelve months following the reading of his book, nine people told me of their near-death experiences. What amazed me was that some of these patients spoke about it without any invitation from me. It was as though they instinctively knew they could trust me with this information. Two had not even told their spouses as they felt their spouse's response would be sceptical.

Presumably, people must have expected me to be sceptical prior to my exposure to his book. If so, their expectations were spot on. This experience taught me the value of an open mind. Prior to reading Moody's book, I must have closed my mind to information like this because it did not fit with my conception of reality.

After-Death Communication

As science ignores the existence of the soul, the subject of communication with the dead remains a controversial subject. Reports of such happenings are treated with scepticism despite the acceptance of such communication by most ancient cultures.

The British Society for Psychical Research, which formed in the late nineteenth century, was the exception, being a scientific organisation prepared to investigate such paranormal phenomena. At that time, there was an interest in séances using mediums. William James (1842-1910), one of the founding fathers of psychology, attended many séances as part of his research. My own interest in the subject has led me to visit people who describe themselves as 'channels.' They have given me messages that they say came from deceased relatives. I have found the messages to be consistent with the characteristics of the deceased person. I also found the communications helpful, thought-provoking, and sometimes quite unexpected.

Yet, because such messages are coming through a channel, there is the potential for the message to be distorted, especially if they speak of the future.

Bill Guggenheim's research

In 1977, Bill Guggenheim heard the voice of his deceased father telling him to "go to the pool." When he got there, he found his eighteen-month-old son drowning. This episode inspired him to look for people who had received direct, spontaneous contacts from the deceased (i.e., contact unsought by the recipient and involving no medium or channel). From the United States and Canada, he collected 3,300 such experiences and estimated a further five thousand in workshops he conducted worldwide.[9]

Recipients of these contacts recognised the deceased in a variety of ways. Some saw the deceased. Others heard words or smelled a particular fragrance associated with the deceased. The most common was a sense of feeling the presence of a deceased loved one. Over the last thirty years, I have routinely asked my widowed patients if they have felt any sense of their spouses' presence. More often than not, the answer is yes—and frequently a resounding yes. They can sometimes describe the time of the deceased's arrival and departure. When it does occur, it greatly helps the grieving process.

A common time for such communication is when recipients are themselves dying. In Bill Guggenheim's study, some dying patients were observed speaking to an invisible being. When asked whom they were addressing, those well enough to answer said it was somebody they were very close to, someone who had come to escort them to the light.[10]

A personal anecdote

My own father spent most of his last four days of life in a coma. Two days before his death, he had a brief period of consciousness and lucidity. I was fortunate to be there alone with him at the time. In the middle of a pleasant chat, he suddenly stopped the conversation as though listening to someone else. He then predicted a successful outcome to a major problem of mine and advised a course of action that did indeed facilitate success. He never regained consciousness again until the last seconds of his life when he suddenly sat up, opened his eyes, and beamed at someone or something invisible to others in the room with him.

Further research and summary

Dying patients are often in need of medication, especially for pain and nausea, and medications can cause hallucinations. Yet in a study of deathbed visions involving a sample of thirty-five thousand patients near death, it was found there were fewer reports of paranormal experiences among the patients taking narcotics. These experiences were more common among those who were drug-free or those on relatively non-toxic medications.[11]

The impact of such communications is not to be underestimated. Bill and Judy Guggenheim sum it up this way on the After-Death Communication website:

After death communication experiences usually expand one's understanding of life and offer a deeper awareness of life and death. They consistently communicate an essential spiritual message:

"Life and Love are eternal."[12]

Emotional Intelligence

In 1996, Daniel Goleman published a popular and well-researched book entitled *Emotional Intelligence.* He showed that success in life owed more to one's ability to handle emotions than intellectual ability, social class, or any other factor. Whether IQ can be altered with life experience is debatable, but there is no doubt that emotional intelligence, sometimes called EQ, can be enhanced with education and practice.

Emotional intelligence is the capacity to know and capably manage one's feelings as well as the ability to read the feelings of others effectively and deal appropriately with them. There are four aspects to emotional intelligence:

- Emotional literacy: recognizing and communicating emotions
- Emotional connection: connecting with the heart and accessing its messages for intuitive guidance
- Emotional management: healthy expression and containment of emotions
- Empathic relationship skills: dealing appropriately with the needs, concerns, and feelings of others

Emotional intelligence smooths the path of relationships in both the workplace and home. It helps develop character, peace of mind, contentment, an attitude of gratitude, and success in life.[13]

The Heart as a Primary Centre

Mainstream medicine sees the heart primarily as a pump controlled by the brain, responsive to surgical manoeuvres, and ultimately replaceable by transplantation. However, recent research suggests it may be much more.

According to the Institute of Heartmath, a non-profit research and education organisation established in 1991, the heart might indeed be the centre for emotional intelligence. Recent findings include the following:

- It has long been known that the heart functions in the womb before the brain is formed. Scientists do not know what triggers the heartbeat, but they use the word 'autorhythmic' to indicate it is self-initiated from within the heart.[14]
- The heart has its own independent nervous system providing a two-way communication with the brain.[15,16]
- Heart transplants function without any surgical connection of the heart to the recipient's nervous system.[17]
- There are more neural impulses travelling from heart to brain than there are going from brain to heart.[18]
- The heart does not automatically follow orders from the brain but selectively chooses which ones to follow.[19]
- The brain follows messages sent from the heart.[20]
- The heart secretes a hormone called natriuretic factor (ANF), nicknamed the "balancing hormone," which exerts effects throughout the body, especially in the kidneys, adrenals, blood vessels, and regulatory regions of the brain.[21]
- The heart's electromagnetic field is by far the most powerful produced by the body—nearly five thousand times greater in strength than the field produced by the brain. This field permeates every cell in the body.[22]

So there appear to be two centres of intelligence—one in the brain and one in the heart, both in constant communication. While unproven, it seems likely that inner peace, authenticity, and congruity would result when both centres are in harmony.

In the East, the heart has long been considered to be the centre for love and emotion, a philosophy endorsed by poets throughout the ages. Western science may be just catching up with this. It is interesting that when people want to draw attention to themselves, they point to their hearts rather than their heads.

The Positive Purpose of Negative Emotions

Whilst there is a vast array of negative emotions clustered under the general heading of fear, there are three negative emotions referred to as 'primary emotions.' These are fear, sadness, and anger, and there seems good reason to believe they have a benign purpose.

1. Fear

Fear is an emotion built into the human condition as a protection. It warns of danger. At one level, it keeps people safe. It tells them not to run across motorways, enter fires, or jump off high buildings. Survival depends upon listening to these fears and following them.

At a less life-threatening level are fears of public speaking, parachuting, and relaying bad news to people. These are examples of fears that are more challenging than protective. The person who feels the fear but pushes on despite the anxiety, gains in self-respect and self-esteem. Such fears present an opportunity to show courage. So in a sense, the fear provides the necessary opposition to enable courage to be demonstrated. As such, it acts as a stimulus to personal growth.

Not so benign is a third level of fear that seems more pathological. Fears in the form of panic attacks and phobias are excessive and crippling to the sufferer. Yet evidence from transpersonal psychology, hypnosis, and emotional release therapies suggests this level of fear may arise from fears that have been incompletely resolved. It has been found that when people experience past traumas in an altered state of consciousness, confront the fears, and go through all the emotions associated with the experience, the phobias disappear.[23]

2. Anger

Anger is also a protective emotion that propels one to say no to invasion of one's person, territory, or reputation. Anger may spontaneously arise to prevent invasion in much the same way the roar of a lioness protects her cubs. Alternatively, it may arise after the event to discourage a repeat of the incursion. In the absence of an obvious culprit, anger can serve as an emotional release allowing one to more fully experience the frustration and disappointment. In all these forms, anger is a healthy response to the vicissitudes of life.

Anger becomes unhealthy when it is judged, suppressed, or warehoused. Holding back anger in order to be polite or socially acceptable leaves the energy stored within. If not acknowledged and released safely, the anger can erupt as rage, which is much harder to control. Uncontrolled rage all too frequently results in aggression and violence.

Anger also becomes unhealthy when it is allowed to fester. When anger is harboured, it becomes resentment. I well recall having a few drinks with a middle-aged Irishman. As we became more inebriated, he started cursing and swearing about "bloody Olly" and "King Billy." At the time, I thought they were nicknames for old mates who had let him down. Later, it became clear he was talking about Oliver Cromwell and King William of Orange. The resentment was more than three hundred years old!

3. Sadness

Sadness is a natural and healthy response to the loss of someone or something important in one's life. Tears may be uncomfortable, especially in public, but they have a healing effect. Grief allows an emotional adjustment to the loss, especially the loss of a loved one. It is about bidding farewell and being able to move on with life.

When I was a child, it was the custom to spare children the sadness of viewing the body of a deceased loved one. While the whole family would attend the funeral service, attendance at the actual burial or cremation process was limited to adult males only. As medical students, we were encouraged to reduce our patient's anxiety by withholding the diagnosis of incurable cancer from them.

Subsequent research showed all these practices restricted people's capacity to grieve. Reluctance or inability to grieve a loss warehouses the sadness, which can lead to depression. With increased public awareness of the importance of adequate grieving, all these practices have given way to a more honest and open approach. In fact, the openness has even extended to acceptance of weeping in public. Here in Australia, we have witnessed sporting captains and prime ministers weep on television. The response from the public to these displays of emotion has been generally positive.

Summing up

In summary, primary negative emotions seem an appropriate way to deal with fear and disappointment in life. In their natural state, these emotions are energies that pass quickly through the body. This can be seen best in babies who can scream loudly and then break into a beaming smile seconds later.

What seems to create problems in the emotional field is judgement and suppression. When trespasses are judged as unforgivable, then they remain unforgiven. The energy of anger and resentment remain within people who continue to view themselves as victims. When grief is cut short or disallowed, the sadness is stored within, where it can fester into depression. When fear is not dealt with, it can grow and become an anxiety state or a phobia.

Emotional Release

Brandon Bays' story

Brandon Bays had been a teacher and practitioner in the field of natural health and well-being for fifteen years. To be told in 1992 that she had a tumour the size of a basketball in her abdomen was embarrassing as well as frightening. Her gynaecologist recommended immediate surgery as the tumour was bleeding and pressing against other organs. Brandon asked for time to try to heal it naturally. The turning point came when a broad-minded oncologist recommended she see Surja, a body-worker who worked with emotions.

While Surja was massaging her, she asked Brandon to visualise her tumour. As Brandon looked at a very dark part of the tumour, she felt intense fear, and the memory of a trauma from her childhood came to her. She had been aware of the episode, and her intellect told her she had long since dealt with it and it was not a big deal. Surja would not let her get away with her rationalisations and suggested she just go with the experience. What surprised Brandon was the intensity of the emotions felt by her four-year-old self. She also realised she had not been allowed to show her true feelings at that time. Surja encouraged her to visualise herself expressing all her true feelings to her parents around a campfire. After she had unloaded all her negative emotions, she became aware of her parents' feelings at the time and felt deep compassion for their pain. Brandon's sister had drowned at the age of four. At times the inexpressible anger of the parents was misdirected at the other children. She forgave her parents. As the tears flowed, she felt a deep sense of completion and peace followed by a palpable energy coursing through her body. From that moment, her tumour started to subside. Six and a half weeks after the diagnosis, she was pronounced tumour-free, having had no surgery or medication at all.[24]

Emotional release therapies

Practitioners who work in the area of emotional release have found a layered pattern to stored emotions. When people enter altered states, they may experience anger and go through a cathartic process of releasing the anger, complete with expletives and pillow-pounding. When their anger is exhausted, they may find sadness underlying the anger. When they have shed tears and expressed their grief, they might become aware of a deep fear gripping them. By exploring the fear and giving it expression, they might then reach a state of resolution. The process often involves forgiving one's self or others. Nicholas De Castella, who has done this work for twenty-five years, calls this state of resolution "reaching one's essence."[25]

This "essence" is also referred to as "one's true nature." The feelings described by people when they reach this state vary, but the most common words used are "peace, joy, love, fulfilment, gratitude, happiness, and a sense of flow or spaciousness." There are a number of therapeutic techniques that help people enter altered states of consciousness. I have experienced three of them: breathwork, hypnosis, and journey work, the latter being the process taught by Brandon Bays. Yet before I had ever heard of these treatment modalities, I spontaneously went through the same process in the most profound experience of my life.

A personal anecdote

My first wife, Nikki, was born with a hereditary disposition to lung disease because of an enzyme deficiency. By the time her emphysema was diagnosed, she had been smoking for eighteen years. Her lung function was severely depleted, and her downhill course was medically irreversible. Even the dramatic intervention of heart and lung transplantations was not available for her at that time, so her health pushed us to a joint exploration of alternative therapies.

When she died in 1987, aged forty, in an asthma attack at 4:00 a.m., it still came as a shock. I realised I had been in denial. The possibility of her dying had been too painful to look at honestly. I had been trusting in miraculous healing while at the same time turning a blind eye to the obvious evidence of physical deterioration. When the grief burst forth, it was more intense than anything I had ever experienced before or since. Having to break the news to our three children intensified the grief.

Grief and sadness ultimately gave way to a plethora of other emotions. There was anger at God for taking Nikki. There was anger at Nikki herself for leaving. These outbursts paled into insignificance compared to the anger I had in store for myself. I was furious at myself for letting her die, for not doing enough to help her heal, and for not making her life happier and less stressful. I felt guilt at being such a useless doctor and healer as well as a useless husband and father. I felt envy at all my friends and associates who had normal families. There was much fear about my coping ability—fear about being unable to manage a home and children without Nikki's help. Missing her so badly, I could not envisage coping with life at all. As the fear became more intense, it would shift back into anger at the doctors and healers who had failed, especially the biggest failure of them all—myself. There was a maelstrom of shifting emotions, all of which seemed to bring intense feelings and judgements.

Yet around four o'clock the following morning, I awoke from a very brief sleep to a deep silence. The house was so quiet I wanted to meditate. Although I was not aware of any vision, voice, or even a presence in the room, I felt a sense of absolute peace. There was a sense that Nikki was okay—a definite knowledge she was at peace, so much happier than her prior state of fighting for breath. In my state of inner peace, I started to see things quite differently. It felt as though nothing had gone wrong. Everything had happened according to some sort of divine plan to which I had not been privy. It had been Nikki's time to leave, and I felt she somehow knew it, understood it, and was at peace with it. I was so grateful to have had the privilege of her presence in my life for twenty years. I was grateful she was spared being bedridden and hooked up to oxygen. I was very grateful she died with dignity in her own home and in my arms. I was even grateful for the deluded hope I had held for her being physically healed. That hope had enabled us to live as normal a life as was possible in the circumstances. Now thirty-four years later, this sense of peace about her departure has never left me. It was the moment I understood the meaning of the expression "*a peace that passes understanding.*"

Summary

Both emotional release therapies and NDEs suggest that the essence of humanity—its true nature—is love. The emotional states accompanying love are joy, peace, and gratitude. Primary negative emotions, such as fear, anger, and sadness, are energies essential for the preservation of the ego. Hence, they have a positive function in life on earth. They protect the ego. They also form peptides that create the bodily expressions of fear, sadness, and anger. Providing these negative emotions are allowed to run their course, they cause no problems, but if they are judged, suppressed, or stored up, they interfere with the energy flow, which can ultimately result in disease.

Emotional release therapy highlights another important issue. Spiritual teachings, especially those of exoteric religions, stress being "good, loving, and forgiving." While such advice is obviously appropriate, it seems more important to be *authentic.* Trying to be loving and forgiving toward somebody when one is actually furious at them is suppressing one's truth. Not only does it not work, but it stores the anger within, where it can fester into resentment. Honesty demands that truth be acknowledged and embraced within, the emphasis on the word 'within.' Expressing anger at another person is rarely helpful and more often creates tension between people. Once anger and resentment have been owned, acknowledged, and expressed in a safe environment, love and forgiveness can emerge spontaneously. Love and harmony is the true essence of humanity underlying the negative emotions.

When one's true essence does emerge, the situation is usually seen from a different perspective. A silver lining in the dark cloud can become visible. Forgiveness comes more easily. Not only can they forgive, but sometimes can even be grateful for the unpleasant experience. True forgiveness at this level recognises there is really nothing to forgive. True forgiveness also gives them an opportunity to become one with their true essence as unconditional love. Then they can arise like the phoenix from the ashes of devastation.

The shift toward God as love

When my son attended my old school, his religious education was unrecognisable from the hell, fire, and damnation of my era. Gone were the old certainties, and in their place was a focus on God as love.

The contradiction with respect to love and punishment seemed to be finding resolution by simply ignoring the existence of hell and purgatory. While such places might still exist in the theology of the Catholic church, the preaching of hell and purgatory has given way to a greater emphasis on God as love. One could say the fires of hell are on the back-burner! At a papal audience in 1999, Pope John Paul was quoted as saying the following:

> *Hell does not exist as a place but as a situation in which one finds one's self after freely and definitively withdrawing from God, the source of life and joy. People must be very careful in interpreting the biblical descriptions of hell— "the indistinguishable fire" and "the burning oven." These are symbolic and metaphorical, indicating the complete frustration and vacuity of a life without God.*[26]

My experience around Nikki's death gave meaning to these words. My initial reaction to her death left me in hell. I was burning up with anger, frustration, sadness, and guilt. It was the worst experience of my life. I felt abandoned. Love had gone. Yet when the emotions had been expressed and exhausted, the whole scene was transformed. I was able to view her death and everything associated with it in a totally different light. Love had never gone away at all. I had been surrounded by love all the time. In my private hell, I had been incapable of seeing it. Indeed, I had not been seeing things as they were. I had been seeing things as I was.

CHAPTER 15

Love And Healing In
The New Paradigm

While the treatment and cure of disease may remain in the realms of science and the intellect, healing cannot. Healing is 'becoming whole' and is about reconnecting the individual to the harmony of the universe. As such, healing brings us to the ultimate mystery of life itself. The word most associated with healing is love—unconditional love

The subtitle of this book highlights the importance of love in health care. The purpose of this work has been to show the following:

- love as fundamental to the art of mainstream medicine.
- love as having some scientific validation in the mainstream.
- love as vital in the practice of alternative medicine.
- love as the essential core of holistic and integrative medicine.

A course in miracles

In the mid-seventies a book called *A Course in Miracles* was published. The author remained in the shadows as she saw herself more as a transcriber for wisdom from a higher source. An introductory paragraph summed up the course:

The course does not aim at teaching the meaning of love, for that is beyond what can be taught. It does aim, however, at removing the blocks to the awareness of love's presence, which is your natural inheritance. The opposite of love is fear, but what is all-encompassing can have no opposite.[1]

My understanding of the course in miracles goes like this:

- The nature of God is unconditional love.
- Because God is infinite and eternal, love is present at all times in all places. Love is the essential reality of life everywhere.
- Anything not love is an illusion.
- Love dwells within us. Love is what we are.
- Love may be hidden, but love can never be absent.
- Fear is what we learn here on earth, but it is unreal, an illusion.
- Life on earth is about unlearning fear and accepting love back into our hearts.
- So love is our reality and our purpose on earth.

Despite being written in Christian terminology, its appeal crossed religious boundaries. Tara Singh, a Sikh, and Marianne Williamson, who comes from a Jewish background, wrote books expounding the course.

Attitudinal healing

Also with a Jewish upbringing, Dr Jerry Jampolsky came across *A Course in Miracles* at a time of crisis. Inspired by the principles of the course, he established the International Centre for Attitudinal Healing, a centre for children and adults with cancer and other life-threatening illnesses. I had lunch with Jerry and his wife Diane some years ago and found them to be one of the most relaxed and inspiring couples I've ever met.

THE EAGLE'S WAY

Jerry finished his autobiography with these words, which affirmed the importance of love not only in health care but in the totality of life:

Whatever the question is, love is the answer
Whatever the problem is, love is the answer
Whatever the fear is, love is the answer
Whatever the illness is, love is the answer
Whatever the pain is, love is the answer
Love is the answer no matter what
Because love is all there is.[2]

Fear as illusion

Seeing three patients healed of seemingly incurable diseases in 1980 lead me to read all I could find on the subject of spiritual healing. Works written between 1940 and 1960 by a range of authors stressed the importance of visualising the true identity of people. They saw their clients as beings of love, light and consciousness. Being able to hold this vision allowed the illusion of disease to drop away.[3]

In 1995, Neale Donald Walsh published the first of a trilogy of bestsellers entitled *Conversations with God*. In question and answer form, he channelled wisdom from a deep source within him. What emerged was a God who loves all creation unconditionally, and who is indeed the life force of all creation. Fear was an illusion to which he gave a mnemonic *"False Evidence Appearing Real."*[4]

What these writers were expressing was in accord with ancient wisdom. Consciousness and love are infinite and eternal. Love is the quality of consciousness from which the visible universe is created. The separate ego is an illusion. Fear and its allied negative beliefs and emotions belong to the separate ego. As such they are illusory, albeit a powerful and persuasive illusion.

In this physical world, creatures are not safe. So they all have built-in software to help them survive and procreate. Even a single cell organism in a laboratory instinctively moves away from a toxic environment and towards a nutritious one. Plants grow away from shade

DR. PETER L. JOHNSTON

and towards sunlight, and spread their roots to gather nutrients and avoid toxic elements. Animals, birds and marine creatures have strategies to avoid predators. Some have weapons to defend themselves or attack predators. Similarly, humans are gifted with a software package called the ego to help protect their bodies, possessions and reputation. The instinct for self-preservation is part of that software.

The ego is that part of the human mind that sees itself as a separate being. It is an inherent part of being human. Everybody has an ego and for most the population, the ego is the only identity they know. They think they are the ego. Once the ego is established as their sense of self, it seeks to ensure their safety, security, power and pleasure. It issues instructions suggesting how to control its environment to achieve these ends.

The ego wants to win, hates to lose and despises failure. Hence most people accept a constant barrage of thoughts advising them which course to take to achieve security, pleasure and control. This 'voice in the head' leads to goals that can produce happiness. But ego-induced happiness is short lived. After a short break to enjoy the satisfaction of the accomplishment of its goal, the ego is soon issuing instructions for the next desire needing to be achieved. Like a software package, the ego does not grow. Nor can it experience love.

While self-preservation is a basic instinct, it is an ego response. It is possible to respond to life and death situations from one's higher self. We regularly read of people losing their lives trying to save a drowning person, sometimes unknown to them. Their first response comes from love, even though the instinct for self-preservation is still active throughout.

Healing and joy are to be found in this quality of unconditional love. Not in ego desires but in bypassing this voice in the head and finding one's true identity as this higher level of consciousness we call love. Stepping back mentally to observe the antics of the ego mind is what meditation is all about. When we observe our thoughts and feelings from a more detached and non-judgmental perspective, we connect to our true identity.

Paradox

Paradox is defined as "a seemingly absurd or self-contradictory statement or proposition that may in fact be true."[5] Serial killers roam our streets, and tyrants commit genocide. Evil is clearly real to those of us on this planet, yet at the level of spiritual truth, it has no reality.

Spiritual traditions, to some extent reinforced by the new scientific paradigm, bring other paradoxes too. There is but one universal consciousness, but common sense tells us that minds are separate and unique. Quantum physics describes physical matter as a unified field of energy existing everywhere. Yet we see everything as separate. Einstein spoke of a time-space continuum, alerting us to the flexibility of time. Everything happens in the 'eternal present,' yet we see time as a linear progression from past into future. We aim at objectivity in science, yet quantum physics deems true objectivity illusory. In this light, scientific objectivity is just a more objective form of subjectivity.

I struggle with these concepts of separation and unity, time and timelessness, evil and no evil, and subjectivity and objectivity. Intellectually, they conflict, but I sense their truth at another level. Intuition is the link to a world of non-polarity. Perhaps this is the reason the heart can absorb wisdom that the head just cannot digest.

The nature of reality

The new scientific paradigm suggests the existence of a universal consciousness that is intelligent and creative—an energy existing everywhere. Spiritual traditions and mystical literature suggest the prime quality of this universal consciousness and energy is unconditional love.

In near-death experiences, people have described a merging with their essence—an indescribable light that enveloped them in unconditional love. Perhaps the energy of love and consciousness may present as light. Certainly, it is a good metaphor for reality. Darkness is a good metaphor for ignorance—an illusion dispersed by light.

If unconditional love remained the only reality in human life, everyone would love and value themselves and others. Self-esteem would be universally high. Life on earth would be heaven—a veritable Shangri-La. While fear may be illusory, it has a remarkable capacity for creating problems in life, one of which is illness.

The pathway from consciousness to matter

The new scientific paradigm suggests a chain of creativity:

- A single consciousness exists everywhere in time and space.
- Individuals partake of this universal consciousness.
- From consciousness comes a stream of thought, beliefs, intentions and emotions.
- All of these products of consciousness create vibrations or subtle energies that surround and interpenetrate the physical body. There they can be seen as "an aura," an energy field capable of being detected by technology.
- These subtle energies ultimately become physical. In the human body, the energies become peptides that are building blocks for proteins, which in turn build the physical body. As Candace Pert put it, "*The mind becomes the body.*"[6]
- These subtle energies of intention, desire, and belief also extend beyond the body, travelling forth to help create experiences consistent with one's desires and beliefs.[7]

Co-Creating our reality

The relationship between individual minds and the collective unconscious might be compared to small tributaries coming off a great river. The tributaries may take what they want from the stream of wisdom and knowledge flowing past. They can also put a filter on the stream so they can block information, archetypes, and energies that feel uncomfortable or unacceptable.

Individuals can take what they want from the universal mind and create with it. Being one with the creative force of life carries enormous power. Desires and intentions bring about events, relationships, and material creations.

As consciousness becomes human thought, it enters a very busy arena. The average person produces thousands of thoughts every day, all with creative potential. However, thoughts held with the most emotional intensity are the ones likely to manifest.

Conflict between conscious goals

Intentions may cancel each other. When I play golf, I want to play well, be competitive, and record a good score. Yet if I do play well, my handicap gets reduced, and I become less competitive, so I don't want to play too well. Having mixed intentions like these usually result in a poor to mediocre score.

"Energy follows thought" is the primary principle of yoga. It expresses the vital truth that energy and power follow the direction of our thoughts and intentions. Where we put our attention is vital. The key to success lies in directing our focus and attention toward our desires and purpose. Frequently, people focus on what they do not want. A focus on illness, even an intense hatred of illness, is still a focus on illness. So it tends to generate more illness. The challenge for the individual is to take the focus away from the illness and visualize a state of vibrant health and maintain that vision until it manifests.

Conflict between conscious and subconscious

Frequently, conscious intention can be negated by unconscious beliefs. A fierce desire for success can be undermined by a subconscious fear of failure. Sometimes it can be a subconscious fear of success. This book has taken me almost ten years to write. I was blaming work and family issues for taking up too much of my time until I discovered I was harbouring a subconscious saboteur. A frightened inner child did not want to see me publish a book that could upset people and bring opposition and ridicule. Once I recognised this part of myself, I could understand why the book was taking me so long. My fearful sub-personality was keeping me busy with work and other issues to block the writing.

Because creation follows the strongest intentions and beliefs, the best gauge of progress is results. Outcomes and actions by and large reflect the sum total of our thoughts, beliefs, and intentions—both conscious and subconscious. Actions do indeed speak louder than words. If our intentions are not coming to fruition, it is well worth looking for conflicting beliefs and attitudes.

Many New Age psychology books address these conflicts. They encourage readers to clarify their intent. Provided that there is (a) a clear goal, (b) faith in success, (c) belief the person deserves success, and (d) readiness to do whatever it takes to achieve success, then a positive result is inevitable. Books usually quote successful business-men, politicians, and entrepreneurs as examples.

Conflict between conscious and superconscious

While there is some truth in these principles, I don't see them as guaranteeing success. 'Superconscious' means 'transcending normal consciousness.'[9] It is another word for soul or higher consciousness, but I am using it here to differentiate it from the subconscious. When we learn a new skill like driving a car, our conscious mind is kept busy with absorbing the lessons. However, the subconscious soon takes over many of the tasks, so we can relax behind the wheel, smoking and chatting with our passengers. It also takes care of most of our bodily functions. So the subconscious mind is the servant of humanity. However it can take its orders from either the conscious mind (the personality) or from the superconscious (the soul).

Our souls hold a broader vision than our individual personalities do. If our soul has incarnated with a view to experiencing creativity, power and wealth as a captain of industry, a politician or a professional sportsperson, coaching along the lines of the law of attraction and new-age psychology would be advantageous.

However, the intended path of another soul might be quite different. While most people would like financial prosperity, many are led to poorly remunerated arts and crafts or to caring for handicapped children or incapacitated family members. Others may desire marriage with a strong, competent and prosperous partner only to

THE EAGLE'S WAY

be drawn romantically to needy and dependent people. Others may think they want wealth and abundance. Yet their souls may have little interest in opulence and may be seeking wisdom through the deepest desires of the heart. The Sufi teacher, Hazrat Inayet Khan (1882 – 1927) expressed this conflict in an interesting way.

I asked for strength
And God gave me difficulties to make me strong.
I asked for wisdom
And God gave me problems to learn to solve.
I asked for prosperity
And God gave me a brain and brawn to work.
I asked for courage
And God gave me dangers to overcome.
I asked for love
And God gave me people to help
I asked for favours
And God gave me opportunities.
I received nothing I wanted
I received everything I needed.

This poem highlights the difference between asking for something physical and asking for growth in qualities of the soul. Requests for a new car, the latest video game or a win on the pools usually come from the ego. If the seeker fulfils the aforementioned criteria, the Law of Attraction might bring the desired reward. But if a windfall is likely to take that person away from the direction the soul is trying to lead him, then it's unlikely to happen, no matter how hard one prays or recites affirmations.

Inner contentment comes with being aligned with one's soul purpose. What I've found with my patients is that when they seek their inner purposes they usually find then. It may take some time and it might involve trying and testing various options and discovering what they don't want. Even then, they can frequently see in hindsight why it was necessary to travel the circuitous route. What can be said is that when we are engaged in pursuits that bring us joy

DR. PETER L. JOHNSTON

then we are on the right track. Then luck tends to follow and we attract what we need.

The importance of forgiveness

In the new paradigm, illness is a projection of the ego mind. But so are our judgements. The people we consider obnoxious and detestable may well be loved by their families and admired by others. While we may excuse our hatred and resentment towards someone on the grounds of something they've said or done, the hidden reason is that they carry a trait that we ourselves carry but don't like. In other words we project onto another person the character traits we don't want to own.

As this revised edition of The Eagle's Way was going to print, the US Senate was hearing the impeachment trial of Donald Trump. Leading the prosecution case was Adam Schiff, who eloquently and forensically dissected the president's behaviour. In an interview at the NATO summit, Trump described Schiff as 'a deranged human being. I think he's a very sick man – and he lies'. Given that these words did not seem to fit Adam Schiff, it seems a classic case of projection. And judging from the expression on Donald's face as he made this statement, he believed what he was saying. It was the truth as far as his ego could see.

Judgements of others are projected judgements of ourselves. They are our shadow sides – those characteristics we can't see and don't want to see. Forgiveness is what clears those shadows. But first we have to be prepared to look for them - and this takes courage. We cannot fight shadows. There are only two ways to remove shadows. Bring light into the darkness or remove the obstruction blocking the light. Once we can see our shadow traits, we can own them and deal with them by embracing them and seeing them as a part of our evolution from our fear-based ego to our true identity as love, light and consciousness.

When we do this, we can see there is nothing to forgive. That obnoxious person was in our life to act as a mirror to reflect some-thing we couldn't see about ourselves. Once we realise this, we can embrace our shadow, forgive ourselves and be grateful to that detest-able character who led us to truth. Removing shadows from our lives is true healing. Forgiveness is the single most potent force of love in bringing about healing.

The Nature of Healing

The first area of alternative medicine Nikki and I looked at was spiritual healing. The 'laying on of hands' is probably the oldest form of bio-energetic healing in existence. While it existed well before the first century AD, its most famous exponents belonged to the early Christian era. It seemed to go into hibernation in the second century AD. In the nineteenth century, it started to reappear in the Christian Science movement and spiritualist groups. In the later twentieth century, it appeared under different names. *Reiki* originated in Japan, *Pranic healing* in the Philippines, *Sekhem* from Egypt, and *Therapeutic touch* from Canada.

Case history 1

My introduction to this form of energy healing came in 1980 when a patient suggested I meet her friend Mary. "Mary understands the art of prayer," the patient told me. Soon after I met Mary in 1980, I was sent a referral letter by a cardiologist saying, "Thank you for taking on the care of Olive, a forty-year-old pharmacist. She has severe fibrotic lung disease with associated pulmonary hypertension and tricuspid regurgitation. She is severely cyanotic, and her outlook must be extremely poor. (One or two years at the most.)"

I visited Olive at home where she was connected to a ventilator, receiving oxygen and Ventolin. I was injecting a substance into her vein when I saw a picture of Mother Mary above her bed, which reminded me of Mary. I asked Olive if she believed in spiritual healing. She replied in the negative but said she was prepared to try anything. Olive was the first patient I ever referred to an unconventional health practitioner. A few days later, I received a phone call from the cardiologist letting me know Olive had deteriorated and was not expected to survive the week. "So much for that experiment," I thought.

DR. PETER L. JOHNSTON

Two weeks later, the cardiologist rang again to say Olive had made a remarkable recovery. A month later, he wrote, "Olive is certainly a lot more serene than when I first met her. I'm sure your faith healer has played an important role in this. On examination, her JVP was not elevated, her right heart was less prominent, and no heart murmurs were present. Olive is very well at present, and I'm keeping my fingers crossed.' In early 1981, she returned to work at her pharmacy. In 1983, she moved house, and I never saw her again. However, I met the cardiologist at a social function in 1994 when he told me Olive had died a few months previously. He was not sure about the cause of death but acknowledged her last thirteen years were productive and of a much higher quality than she had experienced through her thirties.

Case history 2

Later, I asked Mary to pray for an infant in intensive care in Queensland. The little one had encephalitis. Although two other children in intensive care had died from encephalitis, this child recovered after what her parents described as a palpable change of atmosphere in the ward in the early hours of the morning. Present in the ward at the time was the mother of another child with an inoperable brain tumour. She sent a message to me to ask for Mary's help. Months after her child received "absent" healing, I heard the mother took the child to his follow-up appointment. Doctors were surprised at the child's generally healthy condition, and they were even more surprised to find no evidence of tumour on a CT scan.

Scientific studies

In 1998, I attended a workshop given by Dr. Daniel Benor, a British psychiatrist with an interest in spiritual healing. Daniel had searched the literature for all studies done on the subject, both hands-on healing and 'distant healing.' He found 131 controlled trials performed on cells, bacteria, plants, animals, and humans. Of these 131 trials, seventy-seven showed statistically significant results. It was a surprise to learn it was one of the best researched areas of alternative medicine.[8]

I was also quite impressed with Kirlian photographs taken in 1970. Kirlian photos are taken with high-voltage radiation. A healer's middle left finger at rest showed light emanating around the edge where the finger impinged on the photographic plate. When the healer was asked to enter a healing state, there was much more light emanating from the same finger—both in quality and quantity.[9]

Dr. Masaru Emoto took water from Fujiwara Dam, froze it, and took photographs of its crystalline structure. Presumably the dam was polluted because its crystalline structure was quite amorphous. However, when the dam water was frozen after one had offered a prayer, a beautiful, symmetrical, hexagonal crystal resulted.[10]

An expanded understanding of healing

When Mary facilitated physical healing in the first three patients I referred to her, I became very excited. With unbounded optimism I could see Mary's spiritual healing capacity as the answer to all my incurable patients, including Nikki. I sent all my chronically ill patients to Mary. She established ongoing meditation classes that evolved into support groups for them. Nikki joined in.

While there was no physical healing for Nikki, there was something profound occurring in another sense. When she died, she was at peace with everyone. The fates of the other patients in Mary's group were similar. I cannot recall any spectacular remissions. They all died, but they died peacefully, with dignity and with compassionate support from their new friends in the group. When I showed my disappointment at the lack of physical healing, Mary told me about the nature of healing by saying, *"Healing is not about prolonging life here on earth. It is all about the soul and its journey. It is not about extending the quantity of life. It is more about expanding the quality of life."*

One of those patients dying of metastatic cancer told me she had lived more fully in the last year with her cancer than she had in the previous fifty-five years of her life. She, more than anybody else, taught me the difference between the length of life and the depth of it.

DR. PETER L. JOHNSTON

Stephen Levine spent years with the terminally ill, including time working with Elisabeth Kubler-Ross. He described death as potentially a great gift. When death is accepted rather than resisted, deeper levels of one's true nature could be reached. Being prepared to increase awareness, compassion and forgiveness for one's self could bring healing. In his view, if a person has become more whole before he or she dies, then healing has occurred.[11]

I had started with the idea that healing was about relief from illness. So the idea of healing being present, even when an illness proceeded unremittingly till death, forced me to expand my ideas of healing and its nature. As Mary had put it, healing of an illness is about the soul's journey. Perhaps physical healing only occurs when it is in the soul's best interest.

How does spiritual healing work?

In the field of hands-on healing, practitioners speak of being a channel for a universal energy that goes by different names like Reiki, Holy Spirit, grace, and prana. What is important to all of them is unconditional love for the client. If a practitioner cannot view the clients with unconditional love and respect and imagine a positive outcome for them, the practitioner is encouraged to refer the clients to another practitioner.

Research has been done in an attempt to understand the nature of the energy involved in healing, especially healing done at a distance. What has become clear is that the qualities of this healing energy do not fit any form of energy currently known to science. Larry Dossey has raised a very interesting possibility. Perhaps the reason scientists cannot find an energy moving between the healer and the recipient might be because the energy is not actually moving. Maybe the energy is already there—the energy is everywhere.[12] Perhaps the universal energy to which they refer is none other than consciousness, and it seems like the primary quality of *consciousness* may be *unconditional love.*

Maybe instant healings and spectacular remissions occur because the sufferers make a sudden reconnection to the truth of their being. At some level, they may realise their true nature as being consciousness and unconditional love. The role of the practitioner is to hold that vision for them. As such, the practitioners are really facilitators rather than healers. The client's healing is an inside job. As clients realise the truth of their being, their disease, which was a projection of their ego (and therefore illusory), falls away.

CHAPTER 16

The Scope Of Health Care

Having shown the need to embrace all health systems, it seems appropriate to give a broad outline of the health systems currently available. Doing so will give an idea of the extensive nature of health-care modalities in the Western world. It will also provide an overview of the extent to which so many of these healing systems have come into prominence in the last forty years. Some are ancient systems from the East, previously ignored by Western science. Others like homeopathy, crystals, and flower essences are old systems being resurrected. Systems like kinesiology and divination cards are new systems derived from ancient healing systems. And some methods are entirely new.

A map of health care

In order to have a means of navigating this large arena of health care, I have drawn a map centred on the causal chain of chronic disease. It starts from the metaphysical perspective of intentions, thoughts, and emotions. Disorder at this level is reflected in the energy field of the body, which is the second layer of the chart. The metaphysical disorder can also manifest at the physical level either in disease or in detectable precursors of disease. These are categories four and three respectively in the chart. Using this order of causality ranging from the subtlest energies down to the densest physical manifestations allows one to see the levels at which disorders of mind and body can be found.

Various methods of diagnosing these disorders are included on the chart. Space does not allow me to include the many forms of treatment on the chart itself, but in the text, all healing systems are listed and each healing modality can be found in the glossary at the back of the book.

This chart is purely a personal aid to understanding a complex situation. It has no pretensions to being an accurate classification of all health-care modalities. Some treatment systems may have been overlooked. Modalities I have included at one level of the causal chain may operate at other levels as well. There are also divination systems and healing modalities that others would consider peripheral to health care.

DR. PETER L. JOHNSTON

CHART OF DISEASE AND HEALTHCARE

TREATMENT	CAUSAL CHAIN	DIAGNOSIS
AREA OF PERSONAL GROWTH	Lack of balance or harmony in Thoughts and beliefs Intentions and desires Emotions and relationships Soul and personality ↓ ↓ If persistent over time ↓ ↓	Counselling, Psychological, Emotional and Spiritual Insights
AREA OF BIOENERGETIC MEDICINE	1. Changes in the energy field in, and around, the body ↓ 2. Reduced immune function ↓ Increased vulnerability to external causes of disease	Clairvoyance Kirlian type photography Kinesiology Intuitive diagnosis Bio-electronic devices
AREA OF PHYSICAL MEDICINE (PRE-CLINICAL)	If causes persist ↓ ↓ 3. Subclinical structural changes in the body	Chinese pulses Nutritional & Pathology tests Live blood analysis Iridology
	If causes persist ↓ ↓ Patients complain of symptoms	Medical history
AREA OF PHYSICAL MEDICINE (PRE-CLINICAL)	If causes persist ↓ Physical signs of established disease	Examination Radiological imaging Pathology tests

Area of personal growth

I have labelled the subtlest realm the *area of personal growth*, but it might equally be described as the "area of metaphysical causation." From the holistic perspective, conflict in this area of thoughts, beliefs, intentions, and emotions is where chronic disease starts. Inner disharmony may be expressed as words, actions, and behaviours.

Some ways of expressing inner disharmony have a direct link with disease. Unsuccessful suicide attempts using violent methods or ingestion of corrosive substances can cause serious damage to the body. Substance abuse as a way of dealing with inner conflict can lead to addiction. Addictions to alcohol and drugs lead to physical and mental disease, while smoking is linked to a range of physical diseases.

However, inner conflict can create disease less obviously and directly. Emotional and mental stress has been shown to be a factor in heart disease, peptic ulcers, inflammatory bowel disease, asthma, migraines, thyroid diseases and other chronic ailments. Emotional conflict is a strong component in obesity, which is reaching epidemic proportions in the Western world. Obesity and hypertension are both related to stress and are both important contributors to diabetes, osteoarthritis, and heart disease.

Area of bio-energetic medicine

Chronic inner conflict also brings about changes in subtle energies. These changes can be detected by new technology and by the use of extrasensory perception. This I have called the *area of bio-energetic medicine*. Like the personal growth area, it can be a source of disease prevention as well as treatment. Some writers and practitioners refer to the whole mind-body medical field as 'energy medicine' or 'bio-energetic medicine.' Because everything is energy, this is perfectly valid. However, for purposes of understanding the chain of causality, I am choosing to break the whole into parts. Nevertheless, it is important to stress the fluid boundaries between the various levels. In no way are any of these levels truly separate.

Area of preclinical physical medicine

The *area of preclinical physical medicine* detects physical abnormalities before disease is established. Both conventional and alternative approaches look for preclinical signs as part of preventive medicine.

Area of clinical medicine

Finally, there is end-stage disease, the area where conventional medicine is most valuable. At this stage, clinical examination, pathology tests, or radiological imaging show evidence of disease. This I have called the *area of clinical physical medicine* because at this point in the evolution of disease, there is objective evidence of abnormality in the physical body. This area is not the preserve of the medical profession alone as there are other health-care systems operating at the physical level, but medicine is the most prominent of them.

The value of early treatment

Both mainstream and alternative therapies recognise the value of early treatment, and both look for early signs of disorder and disease. The cure rate for cancer is enhanced by early detection and treatment. Detection and treatment of high blood pressure can prevent strokes. Keeping cholesterol levels within recommended limits has been statistically shown to reduce heart attacks. While alternative practitioners treat established disease, I believe alternative medicine is more valuable before pathological signs are present.

Clarification of the chart

The levels on the chart refer only to the science of health care, not to the art of health care. A surgeon, osteopath, or masseur works scientifically at the level of physical medicine. However, when they treat clients with care and respect and inspire confidence, those practitioners operate at all levels from the most subtle to the most dense.

THE EAGLE'S WAY

Finally, it is important to stress that this chart is looking at the whole picture. This does not mean the health-care systems are holistic.

Health-care systems are not in themselves holistic. Practitioners are holistic. When practitioners explore the mental, emotional, and spiritual aspects of their clients, they are practising holistic medicine, regardless of which systems they use.

Personal Growth

Personal growth has become a growth industry itself over the past few decades. Along with the concept of a personal trainer to help with physical fitness and a financial advisor to help achieve financial health, there are now life coaches to help get one's life in order. The primary role of a life coach is to help people clarify their goals in life and set in motion a plan to achieve those goals.

It sounds quite easy to ask people to set out their goals and devise a strategy to achieve them. In some cases, it might be. More often the task will be quite difficult because of factors unrecognised by the client. A man might pursue success with considerable vigour but fail because of an unconscious belief he does not deserve success. He may become so emotionally stressed when he nears his goal that his performance anxiety sabotages his success.

The issues underlying chronic illness are similar. When there is an inner conflict, it is often unconscious. If people had full clarity about their inner conflicts, their souls would have no need to bring attention to the problems by bringing those issues into their tissues in the form of disease. Something as intrinsically complex and perfect as the human body does not break down without reason. Disease may be understood as the life force seeking expression but being unable to do so other than in a diseased form.

Stress and disease

Inner conflicts are always driven by fear. Many health problems are attributed to stress, but in the context of health, stress means *dis-*

DR. PETER L. JOHNSTON

tress. In physics, stress is defined as pressure or tension being applied to material. When people are being pressured or stretched, they are being pushed to make changes.

The pressure may come from life events, from others, or from within. Doing something new and different may bring some anxiety and fear of the unknown, but if the change is welcome to a person, there may be very little fear at all. This positive stress is called *eu-stress* from the Greek word *eu*, meaning 'well.' Such smooth adaptations to stress enhance one's mental and emotional health. In fact, the lack of eu-stress leads to boredom.

On the other hand, when outside pressures clash with inner purpose, distress results. Pressure from controlling parents will create conflict in their adolescent offspring because the adolescent's inner urge is to become independent.

A husband in love with his wife's best friend will experience considerable pressure to ignore this attraction. There may be external pressures from his wife, his family, his wife's family and their circle of mutual friends. His bank manager or financial advisor may also add their warnings, as nothing depletes finances quite like divorce. Just to add to his pressures, he will have to deal with his internal demons—the guilt of infidelity, the fear of alienating his children, and the shame of disappointing his family and friends. Such pressures create distress.

When work and time pressures exceed the resources of an individual, distress results. Because the stress may be intermittent or gradual, it is unusual for the distress to be in full consciousness. Most of the people I see with burnout and chronic fatigue have only become aware of the problem because they have metaphorically "hit the wall." They are so exhausted physically and mentally that they are incapable of working at all. Part of the reason for their lack of consciousness is a reluctance to look at the issue. For most people, work is essential to pay the mortgage and maintain their standard of living. Work also gives them a sense of purpose and self-esteem. Because they cannot allow themselves to think about not working, they ignore the early warning signals their bodies are giving them. When their bodies completely break down, they can look back and see those early warnings. Part of therapy is teaching them to recognise the early signs to prevent recurrence.

Distress also occurs when there is an inner desire for change but failure to follow it. I see many patients who are bored with their jobs but fear they might not get another job with similar pay if they leave. After counselling, many have left their places of employment and found more satisfying work elsewhere. A few people explored the issue with me but chose to stay at their workplaces. Not long after, they found themselves retrenched. When seen a year or two later, they described their retrenchment as one of the best things that could have happened to them.

Distress, by definition, is distressing. Hence, it is not surprising people prefer not to think about it. To contemplate insoluble problems or painful memories only creates more unhappiness. Putting them "out of mind" does remove them from the conscious mind but not from the unconscious. When there is unresolved fear, guilt, anger, or remorse associated with these situations, the emotions remain in the body.

Gaining insights as the first step in healing

Unearthing these suppressed memories, beliefs, and emotions is very much a part of personal growth and holistic treatment. Finding inner conflicts is about gaining insights to help self-understanding. Unearthing is not just psychological archaeology. The power to change lies in present time only. The past cannot be changed. Nevertheless, unconscious beliefs and suppressed emotions and memories, while they may have originated in the past, are energies active in the present. They are causing impediments to ongoing plans and goals. Psychologists refer to them as 'unfinished business.' They require exploration and resolution. Gaining insights into one's own suppressed emotions, divided goals, addictions, unconscious beliefs, repressed memories, or dysfunctional patterns of behaviour are difficult to do alone. They would not be insights if one could see them clearly. There are many techniques—old and new—that can assist people in this process.

Self-help strategies for gaining insights

Some of these can be done in solitude. Examples include the following:

- Meditation
- Journaling
- Writing with the non-dominant hand
- Affirmations
- Visualisations
- Dream interpretation
- Biofeedback—heartmath being the most recent
- Divination systems

Professional counselling can be very useful in helping people to know themselves. However, non-professional people, such as spouses, partners, parents, and friends, can provide valuable insights. Those who have shared a close relationship over years tend to know their friends' strengths and weaknesses very well. Eastern philosophy praises the art of "impartial self-knowledge" but impartiality toward one's self requires sizeable doses of wisdom, honesty, and courage. To ask a close friend for an honest assessment requires no less courage. Truth can hurt.

Conventional psychotherapies

Professional counselling takes many forms. Mainstream psychiatrists and psychologists offer a number of options. Some of the more popular counselling techniques include the following:

- Psychoanalysis
- Behavioural therapy
- Group therapy
- Cognitive behavioural therapy (CBT)
- Relationship therapy
- Sex therapy
- Hypnotherapy

Newer alternative psychotherapies

The humanistic and holistic movements have led to the creation of many other techniques for self-exploration. These are the names of some of the techniques I have experienced. More detail can be found in the glossary of therapies at the back of the book.

- Transactional analysis
- Humanistic psychology
- Logotherapy
- Primal therapy
- Transpersonal psychology
- Rebirthing
- Gestalt therapy
- Holotropic breathwork
- Psychosynthesis
- Voice dialogue
- Radix body-based psychotherapy
- Twelve-step programs for addiction
- Hakomi
- Body dialogue
- NLP (neuro-linguistic programming)
- EMDR (eye movement desensitisation and reprocessing)
- EFT (emotional freedom technique)
- WHEE (wholistic hybrid of EMDR and EFT)
- Matrix reimprinting
- Journeywork
- Cutting the ties that bind
- Inner child work
- Sandplay
- Imago relationship therapy
- Art therapy
- Thought field therapy (TFT)
- Enneagram
- Luscher colour therapy

The new age and ancient wisdom

Another source of insights comes from ancient sources. *New Age* is a term that arose in the 1960s. The term derives from astrological observations. Roughly every twenty-five thousand years, Earth completes a cycle of the zodiac in a reverse direction. Approximately every 2,100 years, there is a transition from one house of the zodiac to another, bringing with it radical changes in direction and emphasis for the planet. According to this picture, we are in the process of moving from the old age of Pisces into the new age of Aquarius.

While there seems to be uncertainty about the actual time of arrival of the Aquarian age, most agree that we are already seeing some of the expected changes. While the term "New Age" is applied to almost anything mystical or esoteric, the words most applicable to Aquarius are "synthesis and knowledge." It is likely to be an age where divisions between people, races, and religions are broken down.

Authoritarian, dogmatic structures holding these divisions in place are already showing signs of decay. I hope that religion will become more scientific while science will embrace the spiritual, as people become more aware of the unity of consciousness, energy, and matter. The Renaissance signalled a major change in direction, but at the same time, it looked backward to the Greek and Roman cultures for its inspiration. In a similar way, the New Age looks back to the wisdom of ancient cultures for its inspiration. As science has been discovering the unity underlying the diversity of creation, ancient cultures that had a sense of unity in their cosmology are being more closely examined:

- *Shamanism* from Asia
- *Celtic spirituality* from Britain
- *Native American spirituality*, with its *Vision Quests*
- *Buddhism* and *Zen* from Asia
- The *Kabbalah* of Jewish mystical tradition
- The *Dreamtime* of Australian Aborigines
- *Huna* (or Kahuna) spiritual traditions of Hawaii
- *Taoism* of Ancient China

- *Yoga* and *Tantra* from India
- *The mystical traditions* of Ancient Egypt
- *Christian mystic* traditions of Europe
- *Sufi* mystic traditions of Islam

Divination techniques

Another avenue to insights is through the use of divination techniques, many of which are derived from these cultures. These can be used in solitude, but impartiality and objectivity are more easily achieved by utilising a practitioner with expertise. *Divination* is defined as "the practice of divining or seeking knowledge by supernatural means." The idea of using decks of cards, crystal balls, tea leaves, bark off trees, or piles of sticks or stones in order to gain insight and direction in one's life seems superstitious rubbish to the pragmatic Western mind. Yet to ancient cultures, such practices were very important. In ancient times when people sought answers to their important questions, they would consult their oracles, shamans, or witch doctors. They saw these people as consultants to the supernatural. These practitioners would use techniques to help them connect to the "realm of the gods" in order to obtain the answers to their clients' questions. The new paradigm, which postulates connection between all minds, including the collective unconscious, has given some credibility to these ancient practices:

- Astrology
- Numerology
- The Medicine Wheel
- I Ching
- Chinese astrology
- Tarot
- Runes
- Dowsing
- Palmistry
- Channelling

To these can be added a plethora of modern divination cards. Here are just a few:

- Medicine cards based on Native-American totems
- Archetypal charts and cards
- Angel cards
- Inner-child cards

In mentioning divination methods as a diagnostic tool for health care, it is important to differentiate divination for self-understanding and using it to determine the future. The future is always fluid. Predictions are never more than possible outcomes. It is sad to see people taking negative forecasts as though these were set in concrete. Negative predictions can close other options for a person, create fear, and make a negative outcome more likely. Unless there is a clear message as to how to change the outcome, negative prophecies are doing a disservice to the client. Nevertheless, it is only the acceptance of the prediction that gives it power.

The power of insights

Divination in the hands of skilled and caring practitioners can give valuable insights into a person's character in the present. Insights induce change. Once people realise they have inner conflicts or self-destructive processes going on, they start to change them. And change is what brings healing. This is the reason I include divination processes under the umbrella of health care. I have seen people transform their lives after they have gained insights from these sources.

Insight means 'the capacity to gain an accurate and deep intuitive understanding of something.' A practitioner may be able to intuit something about a client during a consultation. Informing the client may be helpful. However, it tends to be even more helpful if the client gains the insight without the prompt. Many of the newer psychotherapies are geared toward helping clients gain insights for themselves. Gestalt, holotropic breathwork, voice dialogue, sandplay, and body dialogue are examples. These techniques lead clients away from their usual mode of consciousness, allowing them to understand less familiar aspects of themselves.

Bio-Energetic Medicine

Bio-energies can be defined as any type of electrical, electromagnetic or subtle energetic force generated by living organisms. All these energies are invisible to the human eye. Some of them can be measured accurately and used in diagnosis. Others are less accessible and more subjective. The latter have been referred to as *subtle energies.*

The energy field surrounding and interpenetrating all living creatures is often referred to as the *aura.* To the viewer, it appears as a light or shimmering energy emanating from the body. Yet it's possible this energy field pre-exists the physical body. The physical body may actually emerge from the energy template.

Robert Becker, an orthopaedic surgeon, was interested in the effect of electrotherapy in healing wounds. He was also very interested in the possibility of regenerating lost parts of the body. He did some work on salamanders, which have the capacity to regrow lost limbs. Then he applied small amounts of negative electrical current to the amputated arm of a rat. Rats do not have the capacity for regeneration, but in this experiment, new growth formed at the amputation site and grew into all the missing structures: bone, muscle, nerves, and tendons, down to the elbow joint.[1]

Becker's experiment is consistent with the concept of a bio-energy capable of directing growth and healing in the physical body. Rupert Sheldrake referred to them as *morphogenic fields.*[2] In this concept the bio-energy acts as a template for physical growth and repair. A single fertilised ovum does not just grow at random. It replicates and differentiates into its specialised organ and tissue cells that then form an incredibly complex, yet integrated structure. This energy body, the aura, could well be the force that shows the cells where and how to grow.

If bio-energy is a precursor and guide to physical growth and healing, its importance to the art and science of healing becomes obvious. It is indeed becoming an important component in both diagnosis and treatment of disease.

Mainstream use of bio-energies

Conventional medicine has been using bio-energetic techniques for diagnosing disease for well over fifty years. The best known include the following:

- Electrocardiograph (ECG)
- Electroencephalograph (EEG)
- Magnetic resonance imaging (MRI)

Conventional medicine and physiotherapy make use of invisible energies, such as ultrasound, microwave, and TENS machines, in their treatments. However, these are not bio-energies as they do not emanate from the body itself.

CAM use of bio-energies

Less well known are the bio-energetic diagnostic techniques of alternative medicine. These all have less precision than the three mentioned above, so their use in health care remains controversial:

- Kirlian photography and its offshoots
- Pulse diagnosis of traditional Chinese medicine
- Bio-electronic devices
- Kinesiology
- Radionics
- Chakra readings
- Dowsing
- Intuitive diagnosis

Bio-energies are used for healing purposes as well as for diagnosis. Using music as an example, Candace Pert believes vibrations can bypass ligands and resonate receptors within the body in much the same way as emotions and drugs. In this way, the whole body resonates, not just the ears.[3] Among the healing therapies are the following:

- Acupuncture and its four offshoots, namely electro acupuncture, laser acupuncture, kinesiology and meridian-based psychotherapies
- Bowen therapy
- Neuro-structural therapy
- Cranial osteopathy
- Chakra balancing
- Reiki
- Pranic healing
- Therapeutic touch
- Homeopathy
- Music therapy, including toning
- Flower essences
- Gem essences
- Crystals
- Electrotherapy
- Lifeline technique

Physical Medicine—Preclinical

Mainstream preclinical diagnostic techniques

At the preclinical level, there are detectable physical signs or tests available to pick up early evidence of abnormalities before patients develop symptoms. Conventional medicine uses the following:

- *Blood pressure monitoring* to prevent cardiovascular diseases, such as heart attack, strokes, and kidney disease.
- *Papanicolou smears* for early detection of cervical cancer and premalignant conditions.

- *Blood lipid monitoring* to prevent cardiovascular disease.
- *Colonoscopy* to detect polyps that, if left in situ, might become cancers.

DR. PETER L. JOHNSTON

Physical Medicine—Preclinical

Mainstream preclinical diagnostic techniques

At the preclinical level, there are detectable physical signs or tests available to pick up early evidence of abnormalities before patients develop symptoms. Conventional medicine uses the following:

- *Blood pressure monitoring* to prevent cardiovascular diseases, such as heart attack, strokes, and kidney disease.
- *Papanicolou smears* for early detection of cervical cancer and premalignant conditions.
- *Blood lipid monitoring* to prevent cardiovascular disease.
- *Colonoscopy* to detect polyps that, if left in situ, might become cancers.
- *Gastroscopy* to detect early tumours or curable peptic ulcers.
- *Glucose monitoring* to detect high or low blood sugar and pre-diabetic states.
- *Mammography* and *ultrasound* for detecting early breast cancer.
- *Bone density testing* for early signs of osteoporosis.

CAM preclinical diagnostic techniques

Alternative medicine has other physical signs and tests for detecting conditions that might lead to illness:

- Iridology
- Reflexology
- Network chiropractic
- Hair analysis for nutritional abnormalities
- Postural integration
- Feldenkrais
- Tongue inspection in traditional Chinese medicine
- Intestinal permeability testing
- Vitamin assays

- Food sensitivity IgG blood tests
- Live blood analysis

Mainstream preclinical therapies

Treatment for preclinical conditions includes medical treatments such as the following:

- *Medications* for lowering blood pressure
- *Diathermy of cervix* for early pathological conditions
- *Ablative therapy* for premalignant carcinoma-in-situ cervix
- *Removal of polyps* that can develop into cancers
- *Lipid-lowering medications*
- *Weight loss programs*
- *Removal of moles* before they can become melanomas
- *Quit programs* for smoking, including *nicotine patches*

CAM preclinical therapies

There are various complementary therapies aimed at preclinical conditions as well:

- Nutritional medicine
- Herbal medicine
- Clinical ecology
- Weight loss programs
- Rolfing and postural integration
- Bio-energetics
- Natural vision (Bates) method

Then there are complementary therapies aimed at improving the general quality of life and preventing illness:

- Aromatherapy
- Macrobiotics and other dietary measures
- Colour therapy

DR. PETER L. JOHNSTON

- Toning
- Yoga asanas
- Qi Gong
- Alexander technique
- Various aerobic exercise regimes
- Tai chi

Physical Medicine—Clinical

Clinical diagnostic methods

Once symptoms and signs of disease are present, accurate diagnosis is sought using these options:

- Careful history-taking
- Physical examination
- Assessing body movements
- Radiology
- Computerised axial tomography (CT scanning)
- Ultrasound imaging
- Magnetic resonance imaging (MRI)
- Nuclear imaging
- Pathology testing (examining body tissue and fluids)
- Endoscopy
- Bone density (for assessing osteoporosis)

Clinical therapies

Treatment regimes in broad categories include the following:

- Surgery
- Pharmaceutical medicines
- Radiotherapy
- Radio-isotope therapy
- Physiotherapy
- Chiropractic

THE EAGLE'S WAY

- Osteopathy
- Herbs—Ayervedic, Chinese, and European
- Nutritional supplements
- Diets—exclusion specific
- Bio-identical hormones
- Detox programs for drug over-dosage and alcohol abuse

Comprehensive Systems

Ayervedic medicine can lay claim to being the oldest holistic medical system on the planet, as its roots go back to the *Rig-veda* texts written around 3000 BC. Vedavyasa, an Indian sage, put into writing the ancient oral wisdom of the time, together with his own mystical insights into the scriptural literature called the *Vedas*. Both yoga and ayerveda are derived from the Vedas. Ayervedic medicine utilises foods, herbs, aromas, mantras, surgery, and lifestyle changes in promoting health. In doing so, it covers metaphysical, bio-energetic, and physical healing.

Traditional Chinese medicine also has a long oral tradition. Illness is understood as a disturbance in the balance of yin and yang, or of the five elements, namely earth, fire, water, metal, and wood. Physical, emotional, and lifestyle issues can all create such disturbances. While herbs treat the physical body, acupuncture works at the bio-energetic level—and more. The *Yellow Emperor's Classic of Medicine*, which was written around the third century BC, puts it this way: "*The principle of yin and yang is the foundation of the entire universe. It underlies everything in creation.*"[4]

Tibetan medicine is another ancient system based on the teachings of the Buddha. Living in accord with spiritual principles according to the eightfold path of Buddhism is central to maintaining health. To the Tibetan, physical, psychological, and spiritual balance is the essence of health. Despite the spiritual focus, careful attention is paid to the physical.

In 1981, I was interested to hear Lobsang Rapgay, the Dalai Lama's physician, describe his procedure for initial consultations. Before he inquired about the presenting problem, he would take in the general characteristics of the patient, look at the tongue, and examine the urine. After he checked a long list of signs, including the movement of bubbles in the urine, he could deduce much about the patient's life, which he would then relay to the patient. When asked by a member of the audience why he didn't just go straight to the problem, he responded by saying this technique gave the patient confidence in the practitioner.

Anthroposophical medicine is a more recent system created by Rudolf Steiner (1861-1925) as a counter to the prevailing mechanistic view of the mainstream medicine of his time. Rather than treating illness as a defect in a physical machine, Steiner, a clairvoyant, saw people as entities made up of body, soul, and spirit. Therapeutic techniques used in anthroposophy include homeopathic remedies, counselling, anthroposophic herbs, art, and a form of dancing called eurythmy.

Summary

Once health care is expanded to include mental, emotional, and spiritual factors, its scope is large. Most of these health-care options have come into the orbit of Western civilisation in the last fifty years. Over the same period conventional medicine has made significant progress especially in the field of surgery. So the health-care frontiers, those fighting disease and those embracing it, are both advancing.

It seems obvious that an integrative approach embracing both streams of health care presents itself as the ideal way of helping people deal with health issues. Whether disease is pre-clinical or clinical, orthodox and alternative approaches both have much to offer.

CHAPTER 17

Holistic Approach To Preventive Health

In the previous chapter, we saw how both conventional and alternative medicine had various approaches to maintaining health and preventing disease. Yet the most effective way of keeping healthy lies not in any health-care system but with each individual. The way in which people live their lives determines their general health to a large extent.

Sigmund Freud once said that there were three great humiliations in human history. The first was Galileo discovering the Earth was not the centre of the universe. The second was Darwin finding that humans were not the centre of creation. The third was his own discovery that humans did not have as much control over their minds as they had thought.[1] To Freud, the conscious mind was frequently captive to subconscious forces, to which he gave names like 'id, superego, libido, and thanatos,' the latter being like a death wish.

In the early twentieth century, J. B. Watson introduced the concept of behavioural psychology, although Pavlov's experiments with dogs remain the most memorable aspect of this discipline. Behavioural psychology became more popular in the 1950s because of the work of B. F. Skinner, who believed the environment to be the crucial factor in human behaviour. His observations were in many ways accurate. He saw people responding in an automatic fashion to particular stimuli. The way they met, greeted, ate, shared, and reacted to criticism owed much to their family of origin and culture. Even in the area of ethics, Skinner did not believe man had an inbuilt conscience. He postulated that mankind had established a social environment conducive to behaving in moral ways.[2]

The Vital Gap

In the mid-twentieth century, these two schools of psychology, Freudian psychoanalysis and behavioural therapy, were dominant. Yet both undermined the concept of free will. Humanistic psychology came to the rescue. For the humanists like Rogers, Maslow, and Frankl, it was the power of choice that separated human beings from the animal kingdom. They saw many who did not react to disaster in the expected manner but chose to respond in ways that were remarkable and inspiring. Rather than seeing humans as automatons reacting to environmental stimuli or subconscious forces, they saw a gap between the stimulus and the response. In this gap lay the opportunity for choice. While people might not be able to choose what happens to them in life, they always have a choice as to how to respond.

There is a gap between a temptation and the enjoyment thereof. I smoked an average of forty cigarettes per day for twenty years. When I felt like having a puff, my response was so automatic it was not uncommon for me to have two and even three cigarettes alight at the same time. When Nikki was diagnosed with emphysema in 1980, we both stopped smoking, and I have never had another cigarette since then. Looking back, I am grateful for the gap between the stimulus of craving a cigarette and actually putting it to my lips. It allowed time to confirm the choice to quit.

Less successful have been my attempts to control angry reactions to computer glitches. Computer programs and printers appear to choose the most inconvenient times to break down, and all too frequently, my composure breaks down with them. Self-help books recommending one to look for the early signs of anger only angered me more because I saw no early signs. By the time I remember I have a choice as to how to respond, I am already absorbed in the process of chastising the computer and printer. Stephen Covey, business consultant and author of the highly acclaimed *The Seven Habits of Highly Effective People*, believes the gap is always there but its size depends on genetic and environmental factors.[3] In my case, I was an impatient child who was prone to the odd temper tantrum. Perhaps years of impatience has reduced the length of the gap. However, even if the gap is only a few milliseconds, I have no doubt it is there because I can minimize and at times completely countermand my customary volatile response.

Stretching

While the automatic response to a stimulus is the easy way to go, it only serves to maintain the status quo. If a person skis down a slope in the same track, that track gets deeper and easier to follow, but harder to break out of. Choosing to respond differently is harder and requires stretching one's self. In this practice of stretching lies the road to growth, and with growth come health and vitality.

Stretching physically

The value of physical exercise in maintaining health is firmly established, regardless of its type, quality, and quantity. Exercise seems to be the only proven preventative for osteoporosis. Stretching exercises increase the range and strength of muscles. Hence, they form an important part of training in competitive sport as well as being a component of yoga and Pilates.

Healthy nutrition also involves stretching. It is easy to fall into unhealthy eating habits, especially when one is busy with work. It's also easy to get into a culinary routine during the week. It requires less planning and creativity. Yet, the human body seems to thrive on variety. Having too much of the same food leads to food intolerances.

The body also requires adequate doses of sleep, rest, and recreation. Yet the demands of work, family, and stretched financial resources can interfere with these needs. Frequently, I have heard people say how much they would love to get away for a holiday but can't do so. To them, it is a pipe dream. It's as though they are unaware that they actually do have a choice—albeit that the choice of a vacation might well stretch their already extended financial resources.

Stretching spiritually

If I had to define spiritual health, my definition would include these three things:

- Living in a state of inner peace and integrity.
- Having a sense of meaning in life.
- Living each day in accordance with one's inner truth and meaning.

Inner truth is unique to each individual. The word 'conscience' is sometimes used as a synonym for inner truth and does carry a similar tone. However, I believe conscience can be formed by external factors, and hence, it may not be an authentic inner urge. Part of my Catholic education strongly advised against using or prescribing oral contraceptives and attending non-Catholic services. As these edicts violated my inner sense of fairness and tolerance, I ignored them.

Ethical decisions are not always so clear-cut. When confusion reigns, I have found the best question to ask is this: "What would be the most loving response in these circumstances?" Sometimes the answer is not the most obvious or expedient option. While inner guidance allowed me to take the obvious path in the aforementioned examples, other situations have required more difficult responses, ranging from refusing to rescue a daughter from financial difficulties to leaving a marriage.

Living in integrity also involves keeping promises. If commitments to others are not honoured, trust is lost. Yet commitments made to one's self are just as important. I have given up making New Year resolutions and serious dietary pledges as I have broken them almost routinely. Smaller, less ambitious goals work better for me. Success gives a warm inner glow and more confidence to push on toward other goals. Commitment to grow and develop as a person involves stretching, but the rewards are commensurate.

When it comes to seeking purpose in one's life, it is worth stretching. Finding passion and enthusiasm improves the quality of life and has a beneficial effect on health—mentally, emotionally and physically.

Stretching mentally

Finding and maintaining a meaningful lifestyle requires intellectual stretching. The ideal is to have an understanding of one's strengths and talents and how they can be utilized in one's occupation and other interests. Study is needed to acquire qualifications—and further study to keep abreast of change. Intellectual knowledge also needs to be grounded in practice and experience, or it just remains academic—and such knowledge is harder to retain. Recent research in neuroplasticity showed that crammed study produces only temporary changes in the brain map, while disciplined and practical application of knowledge brings about more permanent changes in the brain tissue.[4,5,6] The old maxim "use it or lose it" seems to apply to brain tissue.[7] The greater the focus, the more brain cells get involved to help the process. But when interest fades, so does the brain map for that enterprise.[8]

Interest and application bring expertise, creating a positive cycle, whereby passion leads to expertise, which brings success, satisfaction, and continued enthusiasm that leads to continued interest and application.

Stretching emotionally

The ideal state of emotional health is a state of joy and appreciation for life. Yet it also includes a capacity for feeling sad, angry, fearful, and even guilty according to the vicissitudes of life, but you must also be able to process these negative emotions and get back to enjoying life.

Attaining such an ideal does not come easily. It involves a capacity for overcoming losses without remorse, forgoing the opportunity to avenge a slight, forgiving others for negligent or hurtful actions, accepting one's own failures, and working at overcoming

DR. PETER L. JOHNSTON

unwanted automatic emotional reactions like jealousy and aggression. Emotional intelligence improves with application and inner work, but it involves quite a stretch.

Aging and Neuroplasticity

After Gage discovered that new brain cells were being produced throughout life,[9] his team at Salk Laboratories found that physical and mental activity generated more of these new cells and helped sustain brain cells for longer.[8] These findings were consistent with other studies suggesting that education helped sustain brain function.[9] It appears we are less likely to develop dementia the more education we have and the more we maintain physical, social, and mental activity.[10,11,12]

Physical activity does not need to be incredibly vigorous. Simply walking at a good pace stimulates the growth of neurons. While golf and lawn bowls fulfil that criteria, they are not as beneficial as learning a new sport or a new dance. The degree of concentration required to master a new exercise results in a greater number of new brain cells.[13]

In a similar way, mental activity involving genuine concentration is associated with a lower risk for dementia. Reading, writing, playing a musical instrument, learning a new language, or playing board games fulfil these criteria far better than does passively watching television.[14]

Dr. Vaillant, a psychiatrist heading up the largest and longest ongoing study of the human life cycle, concluded, "*Old age is not simply a process of decline and decay. Older people often develop new skills and are often wiser and more socially adept than they were as younger adults. They are actually less prone to depression than younger people and usually do not suffer from incapacitating disease until they get their final illness.*"[15]

Another positive contribution came from research on creativity conducted at Princeton University. While Lehman and Simonton found the ages of thirty-five to fifty-five are the peak of creativity in most fields, people in their sixties and seventies, though tending to work at a slower pace, are as productive as they were in their twenties.[16]

THE EAGLE'S WAY

Holistic Overlap

I have a problem with wheat intolerance. When I ingest foods containing wheat, I suffer heartburn, bloating, flatulence, and fatigue. But with the physical consequences, I feel sluggish and less mentally agile. I find it difficult to remember people's names and where I have put my papers and keys. I become more impatient than usual. I just want to get through tasks rather than enjoy them. Hence, I have less interest in other people's problems, and when they do share their problems, I struggle to show appropriate compassion. When I am in these moods, I am more likely to act in selfish and uncaring ways. So, even though eating wheat is purely a physical phenomenon, its ramifications spread into mental, emotional, and spiritual realms.

When people can find no meaning in their lives, the spiritual vacuum can spill over to involve mental, emotional, and physical aspects of their lives. Working in a job just to take home a pay packet gives little incentive to learn, explore, read, or study. It can lead to boredom, apathy, and depression. Staying in jobs and relationships when one has outgrown them and no longer has any love for them not only leads to stagnation, apathy, and depression but can lead to physical disease, especially diseases of the heart and circulation.

Addiction to drugs, alcohol, and nicotine, with all its associated physical, mental, and emotional complications, occurs more easily in a spiritual vacuum. The most successful methods of combating addiction, including twelve-step programs, incorporate spiritual approaches, helping addicts find meaning and purpose in their lives.

A lack of attention to intellectual growth limits vocational opportunities. For those whose natural talents lie in physical skills, a passion for their craft, trade, or sport is essential. Howard Gardner's research showed a variety of different forms of intelligence. Bodily or kinaesthetic intelligence describes the remarkable skills our indigenous Australians have for playing football. Musical intelligence differs from logical, mathematical intelligence.[17] Yet all require exercising of that intelligence. If not, the lack of mental stretching can leave people exposed to uninspiring careers, which can lead to boredom, depression, and addictions. Many of the patients I have seen with

269

chronic muscular problems in their arms[18] are technicians or computer operators who lack enthusiasm for their jobs.

Finally, emotional issues also flow over. Clarity of thought suffers in the presence of anxiety, frustration, depression, and inner turmoil. Frustration and anger can lead to aggression, vengeance, hatred, or passive resistance, all of which undermine inner peace and integrity. And as mentioned earlier, suppressing or harbouring negative emotions over a long period may lead to physical disease.

Whole Health

Traditional Chinese medicine sees illness as synonymous with stagnation of the life force—the energy they call chi. Stagnation in one aspect of humanity's fourfold nature of body, mind, emotions, and spirit can lead to stagnation in the other three. The new paradigm depicts mind and matter as constantly moving energy. Health is about growing and flowing with the constant movement of life rather than digging in and resisting what it brings.

The World Health Organization defines health as "*a state of complete physical, mental, and social well-being and not merely the absence of disease.*"[19] This definition brings a more vibrant picture of health.

First impressions might suggest that our ability to indulge our appetites and desires when and where we wish is the essence of freedom. Yet this degree of license can lead to the prison of addiction. Indulgence can become a habit, and if the gap between stimulus and response becomes smaller through habitual indulgence, the opportunity for exercising choice becomes more difficult. It is by choosing to delay gratification that people gain mastery over themselves. As people gain in self-mastery and knowledge, new vistas, pleasures, and opportunities open.

Maslow's Ideal of a Healthy Person

Abraham Maslow (1908-70) was the first Western psychologist to study healthy people rather than the mentally ill. He used the word

THE EAGLE'S WAY

'self-actualized' to describe well-adjusted, happy people. He described their characteristics as these:

- Exceptionally healthy personalities, marked by continued personal growth.
- Having an awareness of life as a series of choices—one way leading to personal growth, another way leading to regression.
- Open, spontaneous, and at peace with themselves.
- Tending to bring a sense of naturalness and simplicity to life.
- Comfortable in solitude, yet sensitive and appreciative of others.
- Identification with humanity together with a strong social interest or mission.
- Problem-centred rather than self-centred.
- Willingness to work to make the best of their abilities.
- Having the ability to fully focus on the task at hand.
- Thriving on work but with a ready sense of humour.
- Being conscious of an inner self rather than just listening to parental or cultural beliefs.
- Being honest and able to take responsibility for their attitudes, regardless of the popularity of the positions they take.
- A better balance between polarities. At different times, they could be childlike and mature, conforming and rebellious, or rational and intuitive.
- Being willing to see other people in their best light.
- Tendency to have strong friendships but limited in number.
- A tendency to have "peak" experiences more frequently than others.[20,21,22]

Maslow coined the term *peak experience* to describe joyous, exciting moments that were characterized by feelings of well-being, wonder, and awe. They could bring an awareness of transcendental unity, knowledge of higher truth, an altered perception of the world, one more profound and awe-inspiring than found in normal consciousness. These peaks usually come on suddenly, possibly inspired by intense feelings of love, deep meditation, or absorption in beau-

271

DR. PETER L. JOHNSTON

tiful music, landscapes, or art. They could also appear when people are ill, near death, or under the influence of drugs. His research led him to the conclusion that everybody has a few peak experiences in their lives. However, some took them for granted. Others resisted them, and some suppressed them to the point of believing they did not exist.[23]

I can well recall Jonathan X, who twice got upset with me for reminding him about a near-death experience he had had in his twenties. Yet, when I persisted with the topic, he acknowledged it was an awesome experience and that he had never been afraid of death from that day onward. Nevertheless, he still did not want to think about it.

Peak experiences have the capacity to generate a sense of purpose, a feeling of integration, and an enhanced degree of creativity and empathy. They can leave a permanent mark on an individual. While they are spontaneous events, they appear to lead individuals toward self-actualization. Given their level of importance in the pursuit of happiness, it would seem worthwhile to encourage them, explore them in detail, and remember them.

The impetus for Maslow's research came from his friendship with two people who carried these characteristics of self-actualization. However, critics have felt that Maslow's depiction of human potential is too perfect, unrealistic, and superhuman. They say Maslow found self-actualised people so thin on the ground that he turned to the study of historical figures.[24] Nevertheless, albeit overoptimistic, I have found it helpful.

CHAPTER 18

Complementarity Of Orthodox And Alternative Medicine

While I have classified transpersonal psychotherapies under the heading of personal growth, in the eyes of mainstream medical practitioners, therapies involving the soul are outside the scope of scientific medicine. By definition, alternative medicine is "medical therapy regarded as unorthodox by the medical profession."[1] Hence, all CAM therapies and transpersonal psychotherapies come under the definition of alternative medicine.

Because conventional and alternative medicines offer different approaches to health care and compete for the patronage of clients, they are frequently seen as being in competition with each other. Yet they actually complement each other in a number of ways:

1. In their search for the causes of disease
2. In the levels at which they operate
3. In the patients they attract
4. In the centres of activity
5. In the goal of therapy
6. In evaluating the effectiveness of therapies
7. In seeing the positive and negative sides of illness
8. In the area of responsibility
9. In seeing the macroscopic and microscopic aspects of illness

273

DR. PETER L. JOHNSTON

1. The search for causes of illness

Science, being based on observation and deduction, takes the causes of disease to the level of what is observable. While the limits of observation are those of the electron microscope, by deduction, theories of causality can be extended to the molecular and atomic levels.

Epidemiological studies have also pointed the way to a deeper connection between disease and psychological states. Mainstream medicine acknowledges the role of stress in asthma, migraine, irritable bowel syndrome, peptic ulcer, and to a lesser extent, high blood pressure. There is also acceptance that type-A personalities, with their driven and impatient nature, are more prone to cardiovascular disease.

Alternative medicine aims at bridging this gap between mind, body, emotions, and spirit. It seeks causes beyond the physical dimension—in the less tangible realm of subtle energies, emotions, intentions, thoughts, and beliefs. Transpersonal psychotherapy relates to orthodox medicine like metaphysics relates to physics. Metaphysics speculates on how matter comes into being. Transpersonal psychology and medical metaphysics explore how disease comes into existence.

2. Operating at different levels

Orthodox medicine acts primarily at the physical level. While psychiatry operates at mental and emotional levels, its main therapeutic agents operate at the biochemical level. So it is with this in mind I make the generalisation that conventional medicine aims at treating the physical body. While some alternative therapies like herbs and nutritional supplements are aimed at the physical, most tend to operate at the more subtle levels.

There is also another way in which orthodox and alternative medicines differ in their approaches. In a general sense, conventional medicine seeks to treat the *universal* features of humanity while alternative medicine seeks to treat the *individual* features.

Orthodox medicine is based on research into the human body with an underlying assumption that all humans have fundamentally the same physiology. If a clinical trial shows a drug is effective in the treatment of peptic ulcers, that drug will be marketed on the understanding it will be effective for the population at large. Because peptic ulcers have a similar appearance and pathology in all sufferers, this is a reasonable assumption.

On the other hand, many alternative therapies focus on the differences between people rather than their commonalities. Ten patients with peptic ulcers might individually receive ten different homeopathic remedies and any number of combinations of flower essences. The psychotherapeutic approach would be focused on the individual characteristics of clients and the role of their particular stresses on their digestive systems.

Like most generalisations, there are exceptions on both sides. Orthodox medical practitioners endeavour to adapt their universal remedies to individual needs while alternative practitioners may use herbs for their universal effects on organs. What this does demonstrate is the complementary nature of both the universal and individual approaches.

3. Suiting different patients

With the great advances of the past two centuries, I consider conventional medical treatment to be mandatory for the following problems:

- Acute, life-threatening conditions
- Medical or surgical emergencies
- Complicated midwifery
- Serious infections, such as septicaemia, meningitis, or pneumonia
- Trauma—other than minor abrasions and bruising
- Kidney failure (dialysis)
- Heart failure, cardiac arrhythmias, and malignant hypertension
- Endocrine diseases, such as diabetes and thyrotoxicosis
- Severe pain
- End-stage disease, where organs can be safely removed
- Advanced disease where surgical replacement with grafts or prostheses is possible

In addition, there are other less serious problems best treated conventionally. These include minor infections, ear washouts, minor surgery, and vaccinations.

Alternative medicine, on the other hand, will tend to appeal to:

- Those with problems undiagnosed or unaccepted by conventional medicine (e.g., unexplained weakness, fatigue, or pain and/or chronic fatigue syndrome).
- Those with problems not curable with orthodox medicine (e.g., chronic diseases, such as multiple sclerosis, rheumatoid arthritis, emphysema).
- Those who have problems treatable by orthodox medicine but who are unable or unwilling to undergo the conventional treatment.
- Those with no serious health problems but with an interest in preventive health care, self-help, quality of life, or personal growth.

4. Operating from different anatomical centres

As mentioned earlier, research at the Heartmath Institute established the heart as an independent centre of intelligence, working in harmony with the brain. Mainstream medicine as an intellectual, scientific discipline has a strong mental base, and therefore has its focus in the mind. Alternative medicine is less scientific and more rooted in supportive measures. Its primary focus is in the heart.

Not surprisingly, research showed health to be consistent with a state of harmony between these two centres.[2] But while integration is the goal, it is not a matter of having one dominate the other.

I hear complaints from alternative practitioners about the lack of acceptance of their therapies by the mainstream. Yet it is not appropriate for scientific medicine to lower its standards and accept inadequately proven treatment methods. To do so would be to take medicine back to blood-letting and the snake-oil remedies of the nineteenth century.

THE EAGLE'S WAY

At the same time, it is difficult for heart-centred therapies to conform to the requirements of scientific, mind-centred standards. Nonetheless, where possible, trials confirming the benefits of therapies are to be recommended. Indeed, trials have been conducted showing the benefits of acupuncture and spiritual healing.[3,4,5]

5.   Suiting different goals

Most patients who seek conventional medicine do so in the hope that their problem can be cured, removed, or palliated. Their goal is to restore their health to its pre-disease state. They simply want to get back to normal. Failing this, the goal would be to relieve symptoms in such a way that they can continue to live their lives in as normal a way as possible. Conventional psychiatry aims to help people deal with their psychiatric symptoms so they can return to their homes and cope with normal life. Again, there is the focus on getting back to normal, a state that may equate only to the pre-psychotic state for the particular individual.

Conversely, growth is the model which best describes the alternative approach. Disease, rather than being something to be removed, is seen as a call for growth and change. In the ideal situation, the patient seeks the deeper cause of the problem and makes changes in lifestyle and direction in accordance with the newly acquired wisdom. Hence, the end result is not a return to normality but a transformation to a new higher level of functioning.

While seemingly opposites, these approaches are also complementary. Both are appropriate at different times for the same individual. Patients with metastatic cancer will benefit from alternative therapies that are aimed at helping them hear the inner language of their soul. However, if they are having trouble hearing the language of the outer world, they need their ears washed out or an appointment with an ear, nose, and throat specialist.

DR. PETER L. JOHNSTON

6. Evaluating effectiveness of therapies

Both mainstream and alternative approaches seek to use effective therapies. Mainstream medicine uses clinical trials to gain maximum objectivity in its evaluation of therapies. These trials are usually conducted by researchers in a teaching hospital or by drug companies. Once mainstream doctors have objective evidence from successf clinical trials, they can confidently prescribe medication for their patients. As mentioned earlier, the scientific method seeks truth by using large numbers of patients in clinical trials. In this way, the individual bias for or against a drug is minimised. I call this method the "external pathway" to validation

Many alternative practitioners use what I call the "internal pathway" to validation. They try to access the needs of the clients from the clients themselves. Therapies like breathwork, hypnosis, and sandplay directly access the client's unconscious. Bio-energetic diagnostic systems like *Vega* machines and kinesiology bypass the conscious mind by reading the body's energy patterns. They can give an indication of food intolerances, organ dysfunction, and vitamin and mineral deficiencies. More sophisticated machines like the *Mora* and *Listen* actually organise homeopathic remedies to treat the deficiencies or dysfunctions revealed by the machines.

What conventional and alternative systems have in common is a way of assessing the effectiveness of any treatment. The question all therapists need to ask is this: "Is this therapy working for my client?" If it is not achieving the desired results, then it is time for a change.

7. The Positive and Negative of Disease

Conventional medicine sees disease as a black cloud to be dispersed. Holistic medicine sees the cloud as having a silver lining, as it brings a message the sufferer needs to hear. Notwithstanding the message, it would be fair to assume that patients will see their disease as a black cloud with no saving features. Unless the practitioner understands this and shows compassion for the grief of the patient, it is unlikely

THE EAGLE'S WAY

the therapeutic relationship will last long enough for the therapist to help the client to find the silver lining.

So although these approaches may seem to be at opposite poles, both are necessary. Disease has both positive and negative aspects. Conventional treatment can be life-saving, but if patients stay solely with mainstream management of their chronic disease, they may miss the opportunity for healing. Complementary therapies can facilitate healing but can be inappropriate—and lethal—if used instead of conventional treatment.

8.   Responsibility

The rise of CAM therapies has coincided with an increased accent on self-responsibility for health. This has flowed into conventional medicine, particularly family practice. The old authoritative approach has given way to a more consultative model.

Yet self-responsibility is only possible when the patient is mature, conscious, and functioning intellectually and emotionally. When the patient is very young, mentally impaired, or unconscious, the responsibility for their health lies with the practitioner.

Holistic and CAM therapies stress the need for taking responsibility for one's own trauma as well as disease. As long as one blames another, the power to change lies with the other. Only when people take responsibility for their own problems can they truly assume the power to heal themselves. To this end, forgiving another for assaulting them or accidentally backing the car into them completes the task of taking back responsibility and power into their lives.

Yet experience with emotional release techniques has shown that people need to recognize and express their anger, suffering, and resentment as a means of reaching authentic forgiveness. Hence, victimhood would appear to be an appropriate station along the road to empowerment—but not a place to stay too long.

Life is rarely black-and-white. Individuals are ultimately responsible for their own health, but at times, that may mean surrendering their lives to the skill of their surgeons and anaesthetists. At other times, it may mean taking medication according to the dictates of

279

DR. PETER L. JOHNSTON

their physician. It may also mean playing the victim role and blaming others for their illness or trauma until they have the strength and ability to take full responsibility.

9. Integrating the big and small picture

To use a broad generalisation, mainstream medicine puts its focus on the human body and its components. From the organs and systems down to the intracellular molecules of DNA and RNA, its interest is in the details. Alternative medicine and psychology put their focus on the human within the broader environment of the planet by giving attention to an individual's relationship to work, family, environment, goals, and aspirations. Their focus is the big picture. The two in combination comprehensively cover the field of health.

In a way, the two approaches manifest the two sides of the brain. The work of the left-brain is analysis—perfect for viewing detail. The role of the right-brain is synthesis—ideal for taking in the big picture. Reductionism focuses on the small picture, holism on the big picture. Both are necessary. Although seemingly opposites, they are complementary to each other. Both play a major part in a comprehensive health-care system.

10. Myers-Briggs as a Model of Integration

A popular form of personality testing is the Myers-Briggs classification, based on the work of Carl Jung. People are classified according to four criteria:

1. Extraversion/introversion—as to whether they direct their energy toward the external world or toward the internal world.
2. Sensing/intuition—as to whether information is mainly gathered externally from sensory data or internally via intuition.
3. Thinking/feeling—as to whether information is processed in a logical way or whether feelings dictate decisions.

THE EAGLE'S WAY

4. Judging/perceiving—as to whether people act according to definite plans or whether they improvise and go with the flow.

Mainstream medicine is predominantly extraverted, sensory, thinking, and judging. Its treatments are directed externally. Medical diagnoses are generally made from sensory data and are then processed logically. Diagnostic methods and medical treatments are virtually standard throughout the Western world, so practitioners can judge their peers according to the accepted standards of care.

Alternative therapies, particularly holistic psychotherapies, are mainstream medicine's polar opposites, being introverted, intuitive, feeling, and perceiving. Holistic practitioners encourage their patients to be introverts in seeking the inner causes of disease. They rely on intuition for diagnoses. They also explore feelings and emotions and tend to go with the flow rather than have set therapeutic guidelines.

If ever a system demonstrated the complementary nature of mainstream and alternative therapies, it is the Myers-Briggs. The two systems, while operating according to their own standards, together form a comprehensive system of health care.

CHAPTER 19

Conclusion

When my friend Ken asked me why people were opting to see unqualified practitioners using unproven methods when mainstream medicine had never been so good, he saw it as evidence of a serious backslide in health-care delivery. In fact, he gave the impression it represented the beginning of the end of civilisation as we knew it!

His criticism of unproven remedies and unqualified healers still has some validity, although there have been improvements in the past thirty years. CAM therapists and energy healers appear now to have a better grasp of the basic sciences than they did thirty-five years ago. Universities in Australia are conducting naturopathy courses. There has also been scientific validation for some CAM therapies over that period.[1,2,3,4,5] Nevertheless, objective scientific proof of CAM therapies falls short of the standards demanded of mainstream medicine. So in this sense, my colleague had a point.

Complementary Medicine as a Step Forward

Notwithstanding this, from an overall perspective, complementary therapies and holistic medicine do represent a significant step forward in the evolution of health care. I believe CAM therapies have accentuated six aspects of health care, which were not receiving much attention in mainstream medicine. By doing so, they have enriched the overall quality and variety of health care.

1.   Focus on love

Love and compassion have always been an integral part of health care. The nineteenth-century GP visiting patients in his horse and buggy remains for me the enduring image of the caring practitioner. Nevertheless, I believe the advent of CAM therapies and holistic medicine has brought greater attention to the importance of love.

The primacy of love is expressed well in the vision and principles of the American Holistic Medical Association (AHMA): *"The essence of our vision is unconditional love. Unconditional love is life's most powerful medicine. Physicians strive to adopt an attitude of unconditional love for patients, for themselves, and for other practitioners."*[6]

2.   Focus on consciousness

Consciousness is one arena scientific medicine struggles to investigate successfully as it does not lend itself to impartial observation. Transpersonal psychology and some CAM therapies do explore altered states of consciousness. While objective scientific studies are not available, there are many individual cases on record that cumulatively amount to a substantial body of knowledge.

The Eagle's Way is also about changing the focus of consciousness. Instead of allowing attention to dwell on fighting disease or tackling problems, the eagle's way stresses the need to look beyond the immediate problem and focus attention on health, solutions, and goals.

Before we did the fire walk, we were led to visualize ourselves successfully walking across the hot coals and celebrating on the other side. This was repeated a few times with encouragement to actually feel a sense of elation at having achieved the feat. When it came to my turn to walk, there was a sense of confidence about the outcome, even though there was still an element of fear.

Conquering chronic illness is not dissimilar. In both situations, the focus of attention needs to be on the solution rather than the

DR. PETER L. JOHNSTON

problem. While the fear of illness and negative outcomes may still be present, keeping one's focus and expectations on recovery provides an energetic pathway to health.

When I started in general practice, medical records were kept on small cards that were relatively untidy and inefficient. By the early seventies, most practices in Australia had moved to a new system of folders called the "problem-oriented record system." The system has translated to computers reasonably well, so medical records are generally oriented toward health problems.

However, GPs are now being encouraged to do care plans for patients. These are more solution-oriented and encourage the use of paramedical support and some alternative therapies. Hence, the focus is on taking a team approach to finding solutions. I see care plans as a step toward a solution-oriented record system.

3. Focus on self-responsibility

Self-responsibility has been almost a standard feature of alternative medicine. The increasing awareness of people's ability to co-create their own realities brings the focus and responsibility back to the individual. Mainstream medicine has also experienced significant moves in this direction. As this shift has followed and accompanied the advent and popularity of CAM therapies, alternative medicine may have aided this shift in responsibility.

4. Focus on inner causes of illness

While mainstream medicine has been aware of psychosomatic illness and the mind-body connection, holistic medicine has brought this into sharper focus. With the emphasis on co-creating reality by intentions, beliefs, and emotions, CAM approaches have introduced techniques for increasing awareness and making changes.

THE EAGLE'S WAY

5. Bringing balance back into health care

Mainstream medicine has brought great benefits in health care, quality of life, and extended average life expectancy. Nevertheless, these advances resulted in a mechanised approach to health care, one with considerable emphasis on the left-brain, intellectual, and scientific aspects of health. Alternative medicine with its soul-based psychotherapies and bio-energetic approaches has brought a more heart-centred, right-brain approach to health care. To my mind, this has brought a sense of balance to the field of health care. The term "complementary medicine" seems an apt description of a body of knowledge that falls outside the scientific boundaries of conventional medicine but complements it nonetheless.

6. Health care as a spiritual pathway

While conventional medicine excludes spirituality, alternative medicine embraces it. In this book, the accent has been on utilizing the spiritual dimension in order to enhance health. However, there is a reciprocal relationship between the two. Health issues can be utilized to enhance spirituality.

When life is going smoothly and people feel they have an understanding of it, there is little need for introspection. In fact, there is likely to be opposition, if not outright hostility to new ideas that conflict with existing beliefs. Serious illness or major losses tend to create disruption and disillusionment. Painful as it is, the trauma can break down those belief structures and open the gate to a new understanding, including an awakening to the spiritual nature of the Self. As Kahlil Gibran put it, "Suffering is the breaking of the shell that encloses your understanding. It is the bitter potion by which the physician within you heals your sick self."[7]

This is by no means a new concept. The origins of Western medicine go back to ancient Greece, where the god of healing was Aesclepius. The *staff of Aesclepius*, represented by a snake ascending a wooden staff, became the symbol for medicine. In Eastern philosophy, the Sanskrit word *kundalini* refers to an energy resting at the

285

DR. PETER L. JOHNSTON

base of the spine, an energy coiled like a snake. When spiritual awakening occurs, this *kundalini* energy uncoils and rises up the spine to the crown chakra at the top of the head. According to this interpretation, the staff of Aesclepius represents the role of the physician in helping raise the kundalini (i.e., helping the patient grow spiritually through illness).

The Eagle as a Metaphor for Integrative Medicine

Integrative medicine embraces the use of all methods of healing, both conventional and alternative. Yet there is more to integrative medicine than just an extended range of healing modalities. There are a number of principles involved.

The eagle's way of dealing with storms seems an appropriate metaphor for the holistic approach to health care. To me, however, the eagle seems also to be an apt metaphor for the way in which mainstream and alternative medicine complement each other to provide comprehensive care. The metaphor will be covered under these headings.

1. Love as the healing force
2. Self-responsibility for health
3. Trust in the healing powers of nature
4. Using the "eagle eye"
5. Taking a holistic view
6. Integrating the big picture and the detail
7. Integrating fighting and embracing
8. Education
9. Health care as a pathway to growth

1. Love as the healing force

If it were possible to know the motives of a bird, it does seem apparent that eagles must love soaring to great heights because they keep doing it. They have this inherent ability to fly through dark clouds and rise above storms. It appears that fear of storms does not factor into the life of eagles. They have no need to fight or evade storm clouds, as they know they can come out on top.

Humans have an inherent capacity for healing, which if it can be elicited, may allow them to pass through the dark clouds of illness and come out on top. Being prepared to look directly into the storm with honesty, courage, and confidence can reap dividends, not just in improved health but also in self-understanding and self-confidence.

Courage and honesty are qualities of the heart that come with trust in one's self. Having a practitioner who has compassion and trust in the patient is an important stepping stone along this path.

2. Self-responsibility for health

Eagles build their eyries in high cliffs or tall trees. While they tend toward monogamy, they are otherwise rather unsociable. They do not cluster in groups or fly in formation. They act independently, seemingly devoid of the herd instinct.

In my own experience, I have found that patients with chronic disease who do take responsibility for their own health have generally better outcomes than those who do not. Self-responsible patients ask questions of their practitioners. They demand to know the success rate of suggested treatments and the potential side effects. They refuse to give blind obedience to any therapist and are willing to consult widely in order to get help toward healing. They make the ultimate decision about which treatments they will undertake. Not infrequently, these patients have been described as 'non-compliant' or 'difficult' by their therapists. It is understandable that experts in any field can feel mistrusted or miffed by people who question or ignore their advice, but the outcomes appear to justify the patients' self-reliant attitudes.

3. Trust in the healing powers of nature

A certain amount of trust in natural healing exists in all forms of health care. Conventional medicine relies on nature to heal most

DR. PETER L. JOHNSTON

viral infections, bruises, abrasions, and minor cuts. While surgeons operate and rearrange anatomy, nature is an essential collaborator.

In complementary and holistic medicine, the healing power of nature is given an even greater level of trust. Diseases may be medically incurable, but unconventional approaches treat the patient rather than the disease. From this perspective, healing of the person is always considered possible. As long as there is life, there is hope. Given the optimum environment, people can recover from the most serious, life-threatening diseases.[8] The aim is to provide those optimum conditions to enable the healing potential within the person to emerge. Hippocrates wrote about the *vis medicatrix naturae* in this way: "*Nature heals disease. Inherent mechanisms act automatically . . .*

Much as the reflexes we use in winking the eyelids and moving the tongue, for nature is active without training."[9]

Eagles, in their remote habitats, have little option but to rely on the power of nature to heal. They live their whole lives according to their instincts. Unless they are in captivity, nature is the only physician they know.

4. Using the 'eagle eye'

The eagle has remarkably good vision. Even from a great height and distance, the eagle can still pick up minute details. An eagle can see a moving rabbit from five kilometres away. *Eagle eye* means 'close watch.'[10] We use the adjective *eagle-eyed* to describe someone who is very observant.

The eagle eye has been an important feature of Western medicine. As medical students, we were strongly encouraged to observe our patients carefully. We were frequently reminded of this aphorism: "More mistakes are made by not looking than by not knowing."

Holistic health care is no less demanding of careful and detached observation. With the accent on self-responsibility in health care, the eagle eye is a requisite, not just for the practitioner but also for the client. In order to change dysfunctional beliefs, habits, and attitudes, a client needs to be aware of their existence. As these are not always obvious to the client, there is a need for insight. This involves taking the position of a witness and observing one's own thoughts and feelings as they occur.

5.   Taking a holistic view

While the eagle has the gift of sharp vision, its high-flying capacity also gives it a broad perspective. It has the wide-angle lens to take in the big picture. Only from an elevated perspective can the beauty of the overall design be seen. With increasing height and distance from the earth, the fences, boundaries, and borders become increasingly invisible, and the unity and wholeness of the scene becomes more obvious.

Integrative medicine is designed to encompass the whole person—body, mind, emotions, and spirit. It is the broadness of scope that defines a holistic or integrative practitioner. Holistic practitioners see illness as intricately connected to what is happening in people's lives. They stress the importance of exploring the big picture.

6.   Integrating the big picture and the detail

To use a broad generalisation, mainstream medicine puts its focus on the human body and its components. Its interest is in the detail—the organs, cells, and intracellular chemicals. Holistic medicine focuses on the human within the broader environment of the patient's home, workplace, social settings, and aspirations. Its focus is the big picture. The two in combination cover the field of health comprehensively.

The eagle seems a good metaphor for integrative medicine. It has the sharp, focused vision to see the detail and the capacity of soaring to great heights to grasp the big picture.

7.   Integrating fighting and embracing

While the eagle may embrace the storm and rise above it, it may choose to fight at other times. It is well equipped for fighting with its powerful beak, large wings, and strong talons. Not only does it use its fighting qualities for hunting prey, but it can also use them for sibling rivalry.[11]

DR. PETER L. JOHNSTON

Conventional medicine takes a belligerent attitude to disease while alternative medicine tends to embrace illness. Integrative medicine accepts and utilises all healing methods, whether conventional or alternative, with the understanding that there is a place for all healing methods.

8a. Education

The word 'doctor' derived from the Latin word meaning "teacher." Health practitioners instruct clients on health-related issues, so in that sense, they are teachers and educators.

Education in my schooldays seemed to be an endless round of memorising facts. One frustrated teacher described his role as "the thankless task of trying to stuff information into thick heads." With the abundance of resources now available to access facts, the focus of education has moved toward teaching students how to access data for themselves. They are encouraged to do assignments by using library and Internet resources. In doing so, they have the opportunity to be creative in their own research of a topic.

This approach is closer to the original definition of education. The word *educate* is derived from the Latin *educere*, meaning 'to lead out'. Education is about drawing out knowledge and wisdom from people rather than stuffing knowledge into them.

Holistic medicine exemplifies this approach. Healing is seen as an 'inside job.' The cause of a disease and the best approach to healing it are questions only the patient can answer. The role of a holistic practitioner is to facilitate the emergence of clients' own inner wisdom. No single therapeutic technique suits everybody any more than a single diet suffices. Each person is unique. While certain foods are considered healthy and others toxic, there is always individual variation. The holistic practitioner's role is to help clients find their own direction rather than impose the practitioner's own health-care beliefs on the client.

The way in which eagles educate their young demonstrates the way they trust in the potential of their eaglets to fly. They trust nature will bring forth their potential when the time is right. When the eagle senses the young one is ready to fly, the eaglet is taken up and dropped. The eaglet either flies out of the dive, or it crashes to the earth.

8b. Education by example

In our medical training, we acquired knowledge by study and observing our teachers, some of whom were an inspiration in both their technical skills and their bedside manner. However, we were examined on our capacity for retaining knowledge. Successful completion of our degree course empowered us to hand out advice on diet and lifestyle. We could recommend regular health check-ups for our patients without ever considering the need to follow our own advice. In my first ten years of general practice, I would unashamedly advise all patients with lung disorders to stop smoking while I was sporting a packet of unfiltered cigarettes in one shirt pocket and mentholated cigarettes in the other!

The ideal is to embody the principles being taught—to work with joy, compassion, and enthusiasm but to balance work with adequate doses of play, rest, exercise, sleep, and social life. I believe the greatest asset practitioners can bring to their clients is their own wholeness. This in itself is healing.

Eagles do not carry whiteboards to teach their young to fly. They model it. It is the combination of parental example and trust in the eaglets' potential that leads to the young taking flight.

Using flight as a metaphor for healing, the teacher cannot give the student wings. The power and responsibility for healing and growth lies with the student, but the student can only learn to fly if the instructor takes the student up there.

9. Health care as a pathway to growth

Prior to the invention of aircraft, the eagle was earth's highest flyer. Most religions visualized the home of the gods as being above. The eagle was seen as a symbol of connection to the gods and was a potent symbol for spiritual illumination. In the Native-American culture, the eagle was the symbol for the connection to the *Great Spirit.* To

DR. PETER L. JOHNSTON

the Native-American shamans, eagle feathers are still considered the most sacred of healing tools and are used to "cleanse the auras" of their clients.

The Native-American reverence for the eagle as being close to *Great Spirit* continues in its representation as the national symbol of the United States of America. The American bald eagle has its bald area over the crown of its head. In yoga, it is referred to as the crown *chakra*.

Since the seventh century, the caduceus has also been used to represent medicine. The caduceus shows intertwined snakes rising up a rod to a pair of wings that were believed to be those of an eagle. It was said to represent Hermes, the messenger of the gods. It was used in the Eleusinian mystery schools of ancient Greece and in Kundalini yoga.[12]

I have used the caduceus on the front cover because it conveys the message of this book: *Illness is a message from the gods, calling for a rise in consciousness to a state of love and harmony with one's self—a journey from fear to love.*

CHAPTER 20

The Covid-19 Pandemic

While the focus of *The Eagle's Way* has been chronic disease, the same principle applies to pandemics. I am writing this in New Zealand. Their borders closed the day after I arrived in March, and Australia's the following week. COVID-19 has arrived.

The Conventional Response

COVID-19 is a coronavirus which arose in Wuhan, China. When a young doctor discovered it and raised the alarm, the authorities arrested him for creating unnecessary panic.

This suppression of information cost China the chance to contain the epidemic. Had they acted earlier, tested people, quarantined those affected, and followed up contacts, it might have been possible to halt the spread. As the virus spread to neighbouring countries, they tried to contain it. Hong Kong, Taiwan and Singapore had some initial success but other countries have lacked the facilities or expertise to do likewise.

It's now too late for containment. It is time for mitigation. There is no longer any hope of stopping the disease, which has spread to all continents except Antarctica. Mitigation aims at slowing the spread so that hospitals can cope. In Wuhan, during the phases of the outbreak where the healthcare system was overrun by sheer num-

293

DR. PETER L. JOHNSTON

bers of afflicted, the mortality was 5.8%. In the surrounding areas of Hubei Province, where there were sufficient respirators and medical facilities, the mortality was 0.7%.[1]

The commonest source of infection seems to be inhalation of droplets from an infected person's cough or sneeze – maybe even speech. The virus can survive on certain surfaces. So touching a contaminated surface and then touching one's face may be another source of spread. When viruses spread in epidemics, people respond differently, depending on the efficiency of their defence system. At one extreme people die, while at the other extreme some have no symptoms at all. COVID-19 seems to be showing the same tendency. Because testing has been limited to suspected cases or contacts, we don't know how many people have encountered the virus and had mild or no symptoms.

It is becoming clearer that the mortality rate is relatively high among the older population and those with pre-existing chronic disease. People under forty with no pre-existing illness are showing only 0.2% mortality.[2] This stands in contrast with the Spanish flu, which caused many deaths among people in their twenties.[3]

Most world leaders are following this expert medical advice.

- Social distancing. Keep 1.5 meters away from others.
- Avoid mass gatherings.
- Cough into tissues – or into elbow if tissue is not at hand.
- Wash hands regularly – and for twenty seconds each time.
- Don't shake hands.
- Don't touch your face.
- If you are coughing or suspect you might have the disease,
  (a) Wear a face mask.
  (b) Notify your doctor but do not turn up at the surgery.
  (c) Use drive-by testing if available.

This pandemic is a challenge for humanity to work together as these recommendations will only work if people cooperate.

Chinese authorities claim they've succeeded in mitigating COVID-19 by locking down the whole Hubei Province of sixty mil-

THE EAGLE'S WAY

lion people, and using the army to force cooperation. This may not be as easy in democratic societies.

In the densely populated shanty towns in the major cities of India, Asia, and the third world, isolation may not be possible.

An Alternative View

Up to this point, I have heard no advice being offered publicly by representatives of Holistic or Integrative Medicine. Yet I believe important protective advice is being overlooked. If you have acquired this book while the pandemic is raging, it's possible you've come straight to this chapter. So I need to explain the words, love and fear, as I use them in a general sense.

By far the most prevalent reaction to the pandemic is fear, enhanced by the media and by the extent of the measures being instituted to cope with it. While fear of death dominates in this pandemic there is also fear of the unknown. The thought of being confined to home, cut off from physical contact with friends, extended family, sport and social events is understandably frightening. The possibility of running out of toilet paper and basic foods only adds to it.

It is a human trait to like predictability and control. People will stay in abusive situations rather than risk facing the unknown. Yet if everything was predictable, life would be incredibly boring.

Fear may manifest in the form of anger or resentment at the loss of freedom, grief at the death of a loved one or hatred at the Chinese government. Fear may present as guilt or shame for leaders who've been too slow in providing equipment for healthcare workers. Fear is the basis for all negative emotions. It is fundamental to the software we call the ego. Fear is a protective mechanism which fires off whenever our body, lifestyle or reputation are threatened.

It is fear that causes us to feel stressed. Conventional medicine acknowledges the role of stress in undermining the immune system. Doctors prescribe stress hormones to transplant recipients to suppress their immune system so they won't reject the donor organs. Health practitioners recommend mindfulness and meditation to reduce stress, increase immunity, and prevent illness.

Yet the mainstream medical establishment still considers the mind and body to be separate. It leads them to consider emotions as irrelevant to physical disease. So their advice on managing COVID-19 pertains only to physical precautions.

Fear undermines the immune system and opens the body to invasion from external invaders like viruses. People fighting in the aisles of supermarkets to grab the last few rolls of toilet paper present an uninspiring sight. But their panic is also opening them to the virus. People living in fear of the coronavirus invite it to attack them in the same way people frightened of dogs invite aggression from dogs.

While the immune system is not as robust at eighty as it is in teenage years, it can certainly defend the body against a virus. While the scientific evidence is still accumulating, there are strong grounds for believing stress to be an underlying factor in all chronic illness. While COVID-19 is causing serious illness and death in people with chronic illness, the vast majority of people in this category will survive this pandemic.

At the opposite pole to fear lies love. This book puts the accent on love. But this definition of love includes all positive emotions like joy, happiness, purpose, compassion, courage, trust and peace. Love inspires all the activities we do in service for others and for ourselves. In spiritual terms, God is love. So love is the most powerful force in the universe.

In my late thirties, I read two scientific works about epidemics of cholera and smallpox. The authors questioned the illogical behaviour of microbes. Why did some people who isolated themselves to avoid the contagion still contract the disease? How did some nurses survive after working among diseased patients for months?[4]

My father graduated in medicine early in 1918, expecting to go to the front. But by the time he finished military training, the war ended. So he worked in a public hospital in Western Australia in 1919 and 1920. He told me the wards were full of young people with diphtheria and typhoid. There might also have been the odd case of the Spanish flu as they were the peak years of the pandemic. Had he succumbed to any of those diseases, I wouldn't be here.

I gained a better insight into how he survived when he told me about his experiences in the Second World War. He was a surgeon at the siege of Tobruk. The allies had no aircraft. So the Luftwaffe were free to bomb Tobruk at will. And they did, up to five times a day. He saw it as crucial that he walk slowly and calmly through the wards at all times. Had he dived under a patient's bed to protect himself, it would have created panic among the patients.

His role as a doctor dictated that the needs of his patients came first. He believed if he sustained a direct hit from a German bomb or contracted typhoid, it was his time to go. But fulfilling his role in life gave him a sense of purpose and peace. He slept well at night. He was a relaxed and happy man, my father, eventually dying peacefully at 77.

In 1920, there were no antibiotics to treat the Spanish flu, typhoid or diphtheria. We are facing a similar challenge. We have no weapons to fight the coronavirus. So the strategy is to 'flatten the curve' so the medical system can cope with the casualties.

Yet the eagle's way is still available. It sees the dark cloud of COVID-19 and the darker cloud of fear and panic. But it doesn't focus on them. It focuses on creating a state of inner peace and purpose.

Maintaining such a state enhances the body's defence system, enabling it to shrug off any viral attacks.

Courage is not the absence of fear. It is feeling fear but acting despite it – hence overcoming it. The word 'courage' stems from an old French word 'cor' meaning 'heart'. Courage stems from the heart and is a manifestation of love. Whether one takes courage on behalf of another or for oneself, it represents the triumph of love over fear. Love is the secret weapon. No virus can penetrate the person who lives in a state of peace, integrity and wellbeing, doing what he or she loves doing.

A young Chinese nurse, Zhu Tinigxuan, working at a hospital in Wuhan, said this.

"We are still young ourselves, after all.
So deep down in our hearts, we may feel lost and afraid.
Our family members are worried too.
But as long as we put on the suit, we are not worried anymore."[5]

While it shows her courage and ability to overcome fear, it also shows the importance of that suit and how important it is for governments to support the healthcare teams by giving them the tools to do their jobs. No matter how dedicated they are, if they do not receive appropriate physical protection and enough respirators, it can undermine their trust and allow fear to enter. As the pandemic escalates, they will work long hours and see many people die. It will stretch their resources to breaking point.

Looking for the Silver Lining

Geoff was a high-ranking executive with a multinational company. He lived in a large home in Sydney with his three children. They lacked for nothing. The company paid him well for working seventy hours per week. Suddenly, at 48, he suffered a stroke. By the time he finished rehabilitation, he'd lost his job, income and house. No longer able to work or afford a house in Sydney, he moved with his family to a country town.

We became good friends when he was in his eighties. He described his stroke as the worst event of his life – but his salvation. He had no inkling of what he'd been doing to his body. Once he recovered, he saw things more clearly. He discovered the joys of family life, but regretted being an absentee father through his children's formative years. He soon appreciated the beauty of nature, becoming a landscape artist and an avid gardener. He never regained wealth, but was so happy and proud of his marriage of sixty years. They were close to their children, grandchildren and great-grandchildren. He saw his life after his stroke as much happier than it was prior to it.

Over fifty years in family practice, I've seen many people stop smoking, cut back the booze, lose weight and change their lifestyle after having a heart attack. They can look back at their illnesses and see them as wake-up calls.

The Silver Lining at the Personal Level

I suspect this enforced isolation could have a similar benefit for many people. Their first thoughts might be; "this shouldn't be happening. It's not fair. I'm not going along with all this." Yet this attitude is only fighting reality, which always creates more pain. I'm sure most people will eventually adjust to this new reality.

Eastern philosophy speaks of *enlightenment*. It is a state of mind where one totally trusts that a benign and loving force governs life. Enlightened beings know that behind the appearance of disaster lies a loving purpose. So, rather than say 'my way or the highway', they say 'thy will be done'. Their attitude allows them to be happy regardless of what is happening in the world. Paul of Tarsus described this state as *the peace of God that passeth understanding*.[6] John the evangelist wrote of *being in the world, but not of it*.[7] Because no earthly event can upset this state of joy, it is indestructible. This state of enlightenment is the ultimate goal of human endeavour. In symbolic terms, it is the butterfly status that caterpillars are destined to become.

This period of isolation can be the cocoon wherein we go inside to find this state of joy. To listen to the voice of love which comes to us via feelings, intuition, dreams, meditation, instincts and interest in people, nature, pets, games and life itself.

It's about taking time out from the voice in our head, that fear-laden yapping, indefatigable commentator telling us what to do and castigating us for our minor errors. Now we have less distractions, it's a good time to allow all our unexpressed emotions to surface. To heal the wounds of the past and repair dysfunctional relationships. To forgive our enemies and ourselves. These are the steps that help us clean the windscreens that distort our capacity to see the truth about life.

With the future more unpredictable than usual, it's a good time to live in the present. To look at the talents or interests we've put on the back burner because of the busy lives we've been leading. Maybe it's time to get out the musical instrument, the pastels, cook new recipes, play board games with the kids? As Neale Donald Walsch wrote in Conversations with God:

DR. PETER L. JOHNSTON

If you don't go within, you'll go without.[8]

It's also a good time to reflect on what is important in life. Does the extra income we earn by living overseas outweigh the benefit of being around extended family and childhood friends? Having just been stood down from my job, do I really want to return to that type of work? Now I'm at home with the kids, do I want to escape back into a job as soon as I can? Or do I want to stay home and be a full-time mum? Have I got talents that are not being developed or utilised? Can I sit around reading and playing games without feeling guilty for wasting time?

If I were to issue some holistic instructions, they might go like this.

- Use the word 'spatial distancing' - not social distancing. Keep up connections by phone, email, and social media.
- Use the time in isolation to reflect, contemplate, read uplifting books, share jokes online, watch comedies and deepen the connection with those sharing your quarantine.
- Limit exposure to the media to reduce the negativity.
- Where possible, go to parks, beaches, forests and gardens. Nature can lift your energies and settle your cabin fever.
- Keep your attention in the present moment. Worrying about the future is what creates fear.
- Accept isolation for the time it takes to flatten the curve. It helps the vulnerable and supports healthcare personnel.
- Remember that joy is an inside job. Going inside physically is an opportunity to go inside your heart and find it.
- And a message:

The coronavirus COVID19 is infectious – but fear is also infectious.
In the absence of fear, the coronavirus cannot gain a foothold.
It is fear that cripples our body's immune system and by doing so,
opens the gate to microscopic invaders like the corona virus.
Now is the time to truly know, and trust, that our defence system
has the power and know-how to see off any invader

The Silver Lining at the Global Level

It's worth looking at the state of our world before COVID-19 came into view:

- Old-growth forests, the lungs of the Earth, were being destroyed in the Amazon basin by fire and deforestation.[9]
- After a long drought, bush fires in Australia destroyed an estimated 20% of Australia's forests, along with millions of native animals.[10]
- Melting of ice in Greenland and the Arctic were causing a rise in sea-levels and considerable concern for Pacific Islanders.
- Earth's population reached 7.5 billion, aggravating the problems of poverty, starvation and pollution.
- Accommodating this large population was causing the removal of natural habitats for species, some of which were becoming endangered or extinct.
- The gap between rich and poor was widening in Western democracies.
- Israel was increasing its occupation of the West Bank, making peace in the Middle East more elusive.
- USA and China, two of the nine countries with nuclear weapons, were engaged in a trade war.

Since 1947, the Bulletin of the Atomic Scientists has kept a doomsday clock as a symbol of the likelihood of a man-made global catastrophe – represented as midnight. Our safest point came in 1991 when the clock showed 17 minutes to midnight. On 23rd January 2020, the doomsday clock pointed to 1 minute 40 seconds, the closest it has ever come to global catastrophe.[11]

Governments are spending vast amounts of money to cushion the economic consequences of the pandemic and enable a return to normality. It is likely that most countries will have less money and more debt than they had before the pandemic.

With this in mind, after people have spent weeks or months in isolation, reflecting on what is important in life, isn't this going to be a good opportunity for a reset? Will Australians want to spend $80 billion on submarines that won't be ready till 2030, when they are likely to be out of date? Will countries wish to continue spending vast sums on armaments?

Time Magazine's Person of the Year, Greta Thunberg has become the figurehead for a generation of young people acutely aware of the urgency of climate change.

A small opening in the dark clouds has been the amazing extent to which levels of air pollution subsided once factories, planes and cars reduced their toxic exhausts.[12] While it could all go back to where it was once the lockdowns cease, it will strengthen the case for green energy. When those who live in the major cities of Europe and China have experienced easier breathing and seen blue skies for the first time in years, they are likely to be advocates for eliminating fossil fuels.

However, climate change is not the only issue. We have other problems. Pollution of our land, sea and air, poverty, overpopulation and endangered species are evidence of our imbalance with nature. We need cooperation, not competition.

If wealthy nations redirected money spent on defence to easing world poverty, it would transform our world. It would remove much of the incentive for terrorists to attack. It would reduce the need for the poor in Brazil to make money selling timber. Overpopulation occurs mainly in poor countries. When people know their children

THE EAGLE'S WAY

will survive, they have fewer children.[13] Fewer people will bring less pollution. Such a move from fearing our neighbours to caring about them would be revolutionary, serving also to reduce the threat of a nuclear holocaust.

FINAL WORDS

The Eagle's Way is all about seeing the storm but not staying focused on it. The eagle sees storm clouds but goes through them, keeping its focus on getting above them and flying to its desired goal.

At the personal level, the eagle's way is to see the damage COVID-19 is doing, but lift our focus to taking measures that will help others to cope with the storm. And to treat isolation as a retreat – an opportunity to find inner peace.

At the global level, the eagle's way is to elevate our focus above the dark clouds of death and financial disaster being wrought by COVID-19. Then we might see the potential gift in this pandemic. It's the opportunity to visualise a new Earth in which recognition of our common humanity replaces the old divisions. By respecting each other and our planetary home, we can find the unity of purpose to solve our problems and create a golden age here on Earth.

ENDNOTES

Introduction

1   Professor Rob Morrison OAM. Professorial Fellow at Flinders University. *Sydney Morning Herald*, February 4-5, 2012.

2   Bettina Arndt. *The Australian*. Friday, March 2, 2012.

3   Risks and Benefits of Oestrogen Plus Progestin in Healthy Postmenopausal Women. Principal results from the Women's Health Initiative Randomized Control Trial. JAMA 2002: 288(3): 321-323.

4   Daniel Mowrey PhD. *Herbal Tonic Remedies*. Keats Publishing. New Canaan, Connecticut. 1993

5   A 2009 Cochrane review of acupuncture and dry needling for low back pain demonstrated that acupuncture was more effective than placebo.

6   David Taylor—Reilly et al. *Is Evidence for Homeopathy Reproducible?* This study used homeopathically potentized allergens in asthma sufferers and found the results were superior to placebo. Lancet 1994

7   Kanowski S & Hoerr R *Gingko biloba extract EGb 761 in dementia:analyses of a 24 week, multi-center, double-blind placebo-controlled, randomized trial.* Pharmacopsychiatry Nov 2003: 36(6): 297-303

8   K.Linde et al. *St John's Wort for depression. Meta-analysis of randomized controlled trials.* British Journal of Psychiatry 2005. 186: 99-107

305

DR. PETER L. JOHNSTON

9   Dr Daniel Benor. *Survey of Spiritual Healing Research.* Complementary Medical Research Vol 4. Sept 1990: 9-33. He collected 131 studies, mostly non-human, of which 56 showed significant results.

Chapter 1

1   James Le Fanu, *The Rise and Fall of Modern Medicine* (New York: Abacus, 1999).

2   *Office of Health Economics Compendium of Health Statistics, 1984.*

3   Wurtman R. J., Bettiker R. L., *The Slowing of Treatment Discovery 1965-1995*. Nature Medicine 1 (1995): 1122-5.

4   Benkoussan, A. *Complementary Medicine: Where Lies Its Appeal?"* Medical Journal of Australia *170* (1999): 247-8.

5   MacLennan, A. H, Wilson, D. H., Taylor, A. W., *Prevalence and Cost of Alternative Medicine.* Preventive Medicine *35* (2002): 166-73.

6   Cardinal Health, Roy Morgan, market research, 2004.

7   Eisenberg, D., *Unconventional Medicine in the United States.* New England Journal of Medicine *328* (1993): 282-3.

8   Eisenberg, D. M., Davis, R. B., Effner, S. L., et al., *Trends in Alternative Medicine Use in United States 1990-1997.* JAMA 280 (1998): 1569-75.

9   Haustermann, D., *Wachsendes verterauen in naturheilmittel,* Dtsch Arzteblatt *94* (1997): 1857-8.

10   Fisher, P., Ward, A., *Complementary Medicine in Europe.* British Medical Journal 309 (1994): 107-111.

11   Comfrey and tryptophan were removed from sale in Australia. In the United States, the FDA banned the public sale of L-Tryptophan in 1990 and advised manufacturers to remove comfrey products from the market in 2001.

12   Way, B., Stewart, A., Crocker, A., *Usage of Alternative Medicines by Patients Presenting to an Emergency Department,* Emergency Medicine *8* (1996): 5-10.

THE EAGLE'S WAY

13   Bensoussan, A., Myers S., *Towards a Safer Choice: The Practice of Traditional Chinese Medicine in Australia*," Sydney Faculty of Health, University of Western Sydney, 1966.
14   Crook, S., Pakulski, S., Waters, M. *Postmodernization: change in advanced society.* London, Sage, 1992.
15   Concise Oxford Dictionary.
16   ibid.

Chapter 2

1   Traditional Chinese Medicine, Tibetan Medicine and Ayervedic Medicine.
2   MIMS by MediMedia Australia Pty Ltd.
3   ibid.
4   Raphael, C., Ahrens, J., Fowler N. *Financing end-of-life care in the USA.* J. R. Soc Med 2001 Sept 94(9): 458-61.

Chapter 3

1   Luke 6:27-8. Good News Bible. The full quotation makes the message clear:
      "But I tell you who hear me: Love your enemies, do good to those who hate you, bless those who curse you and pray for those who mistreat you."
2   Professor W Lenz. *The History of Thalidomide.* Lecture delivered in 1992 by the doctor who first raised the alarm about the damage it was causing.
3   Medinfo: *Non-Steroidal Anti-Inflammatory Drugs.*
4   *Risks and Benefits of Oestrogen Plus Progestin in Healthy Postmenopausal Women. Principal results from the Women's Health Initiative Randomized Control Trial.* JAMA 2002: 288(3): 321-323.
5   Ralph W. Moss, *Questioning Chemotherapy*, (Brooklyn, New York: Equinox, 1995).
6   Lazarou, J., Pomeranz, B. H., Corey P. N., *Incidence of Drug Reactions in Hospitalized Patients: A Meta-Analysis of Prospective Studies.* Journal of the American Medical Association 279 (1997): 1200-5.

307

DR. PETER L. JOHNSTON

7   Stanfield, B., *Mortality from Iatrogenic Causes*. Journal of the American Medical Association (2000).

8   United Medical Protection Group required a rescue package from the Australian Government in order to survive.

9   Medical Observer, 2001.

10   Schattner and Conan, 1998.

11   Nogrady, B., *Red Flags for Suicidal Doctors*, JAMA 289 (2003): 3161-6.

12   Balarajan 1989, Safinosky 1980, Pitts et al 1979, Schlicht et al 1990.

13   *Kalokerinos v. Burnett.*

Chapter 4

1   Lind, J., *A Treatise of the Scurvy*, 1754.

2   *Encyclopaedia Brittanica*, 2002.

3   *Immunotherapy for cancer.* http://www.cancer-info.com/immuno.htm.

4   Williams, D., *Bitter Pills: Subtitled Dealing with Depression*, TIME Magazine (November 21, 2005): 49.

5   ibid., 50.

6   ibid., 48.

7   *Encyclopaedia of World Mythology* (London: Peerage Books), 140. In Greek mythology, Procrustes was a criminal who had an iron bed to which he took his captives. He was obviously quite obsessive-compulsive, as he liked them to fit his bed. If they were too short they were stretched on the rack; if they were too tall they had a proportion of their legs amputated.

8   Vaughan, F., *The Inward Arc* (Nevada City, CA: Blue Dolphin, 1995), 53.

9   This was a quote hanging in Einstein's office in Princeton. Taken from the collected quotes from Albert Einstein. Compiled by Kevin Harris.

10   Fritjof Capra, *Swimming in the Same Ocean*, in Uncommon Wisdom (Flamingo: HarperCollins, 1989), 127-8.

11   ibid., 422.

12   Jung, C. G. *Memories, Dreams, Reflections.*

13 Elisabeth Kubler-Ross, *On Death and Dying* (New York: Simon and Schuster, 1969).

Chapter 5

1 Benson, H., *Timeless Healing: The Power and Biology of Belief* (New York: Fireside, 1996).

2 Paul's First Letter to the Corinthians 13:13, Good News Bible.

3 O'Regan, B., and Hirschberg, C., *Spontaneous Remission: An Annotated Bibliography* (Sausalito, CA: Institute of Noetic Sciences, 1993).

4 Dr. Ian Gawler. The Five Stages of Hope. Mind, Immunity & Health, 1995.

5 Paul's Epistle to the Hebrews 10:1-2, King James Bible.

6 Pennini B, Guralink J, Pahor M, Ferrucci L, Corhan J, Wallace R.B et al: *Chronically depressed mood and cancer risk in older persons.* J Nat Cancer Inst 1998: 90; 1888-93

7 Masters, S., "Placebo is not a dirty word," *Med Observer (September 13)* 2002.

8 Mosely B, O'Malley K, Petersen N, Menke T, Brody B, Kuykendall D, Hollingsworth J, Ashton C & Wray N. *A controlled trial of arthroscopic surgery for osteoarthritis of the knee.* New England Journal of Medicine 2002; 347:81-88. July 2002

9 Young, Landon, *Oklahoma's Hidden Treasure: From 1941-57.* Wolf studied digestion with the help of Tom Little, a patient with a hole in his stomach from a childhood accident.

10 Fielding, J. W. L., Fagg, S. L., Jones, B. G. et al., "An Interim Report of a Prospective Randomized Controlled Study of Adjuvant Chemotherapy in Operable Gastric Cancer: British Stomach Cancer Group," *World Journal of Surgery 3* (1983): 457-471.

11 Dossey, L., *Healing Words: Subtitled The Power of Prayer and the Practice of Medicine* (New York: HarperCollins, 1993), 135-6.

12 Toone, W. M., "Effects of Vitamin E: Good and Bad," *New England Journal of Medicine 289* (1973): 689-98.

13 Anderson, T. W., "Vitamin E in Angina Pectoris," *Canadian Medical Assoc. Journal 110* (1974): 401-6. Gillian, R., Mondell, B.,

and Warbasse J. R., "Quantitative Evaluation of Vitamin E in the Treatment of Angina Pectoris," *American Heart 93* (1977): 444-9.

14 Uhlenhuth, E. H., Cantor, A., Neustadt, O., and Payson, H. E., "The Symptomatic Relief of Anxiety with Meprobamate, Phenobarbital and Placebo," *American Journal of Psychiatry 115* (1959): 905-10.

15 Eriksson, P., Perfilieva, E., Bjork-Eriksson, T., Alborn, A., Nordborg, C., Peterson, D., and Gage, E., "Neurogenesis in the adult human hippocampus," *Nature Medicine 4* (2011): 1313-17.

16 Doidge Norman, MD, *The Brain That Changes Itself. Revised Edition* (New York: Scribe, 2010), 20-4.

17 Aquilar, M. J., "Recovery of motor function after unilateral infarction of the basis pontis," *American Journal of Physical Medicine 48* (1969): 279-88.

18 Bach-y-Rita, P., Brain plasticity as a basis for therapeutic procedures.

19 Headache Study Group, "Predictors of outcome in headache patients presenting to family physicians. A one-year prospective study *Headache 26* (1996): 285-94.

20 Jospe, M., *The Placebo Effect in Healing* (Toronto: Lexington Books, 1978).

21 Cohen, M., Kotsirilis, V., Bajraskewski, T., and Hassed C. Long. Consultations and quality of care," *JAIMA 19* (2002): 19-22.

22 *Concise Oxford Dictionary.*

23 House, J. S., Landis, K. R., Umberson, D., "Social Relationships and Health," *Science 241* (1988): 540-5.

24 Greenwood, D. C., Muir, K. R., Packham, C. J., et al. "Coronary heart disease: A review of the role of psychosocial stress and social support," *Journal of Public Health Medicine 18* (1996): 221-31.

25 Seeman, T. E., and Syme, S.L. "Social networks and coronary artery disease: A comparison of the structure and function of social relations as predictors of disease," *Psychosomatic Medicine 49* (1987): 341-54.

26 Medalie, J. H., and U. Goldbourt, "Angina pectoris among 10,000 men: and other risk factors as evidenced by a multivar-

THE EAGLE'S WAY

iate analysis of a five-year incidence study," *American Journal of Medicine 60* (1976):

27   Medalie, J. H., Stange, K. C., Zyzanski, S. J., and U. Goldbourt, "The importance of biopsychosocial factors in the development of duodenal ulcer in a cohort of middle-aged men," *American Journal of Epidemiology. 136* (1992): 1280-7.

28   Holmes, T. H., *Multidiscipline studies of tuberculosis. In P. Sparer edition of Personality, Stress and Tuberculosis* (New York: Int. Universities Press, 1956

29   Hoffman, S., and M. C. Hatch, "Stress, social support and pregnancy outcome: A reassessment based on recent research," *Paediatric & Perinatal Epidemiology 10* (1996): 380-405.

30   Boyce, W. T., Schaefer, C., and C. Uitti, "Permanence and Change: psychosocial factors in the outcome of adolescent pregnancy," *Social Science and Medicine 21* (1985): 1279-87.

31   Leserman, J., Jackson, E., Petitto, J., et al., "Progression to AIDS: the effects of stress, depressive symptoms and social support," *Psychosomatic Medicine 61* (1999): 397-406.

32   Russek, L. G., and G. E. Schwartz, "Perceptions of parental caring predict health status in midlife: A 35-year follow-up of the Harvard Mastery of Stress Study," *Psychosomatic Medicine 59* (1997): 144-9.

33   Graves, P. L., Thomas, C. B., and L. A. Mead, "Familial and Psychological Predictors of Cancer," *Cancer Detection & Prevention 15* (1991): 59-64.

34   Lynch, J. J., The Broken Heart: The Medical Consequences of Loneliness (New York: Basic Books, 1977).

35   Medalie, J. H., and Goldbourt, "Angina pectoris among 10,000 men. Psychosocial and other risk factors as evidenced by a multivariate analysis of a five-year incidence study," *American Journal of Medicine 60* (1976): 1280-7.

36   Horsten, M., Kirkeeide, R., Svane, B., Schenck-Gustafsson, K., Blom, M., Wamala, S., and K. Orth-Gomer, "Social support and coronary artery disease in women."

37   Egolf, B., Lasker, J., Wolf, S., and L. Potvin, "Featuring health risks and mortality: the Roseto effect: a 50-year comparison of

DR. PETER L. JOHNSTON

mortality rates," *American Journal of Public Health 82* (1992): 1089-92.

38 Wolf, S., "Predictors of myocardial infarction over a span of 30 years in Roseto, Pennsylvania," *Integrative Physiological & Behavioural Science 27* (1992): 246-57.

39 Friedman, E., Katcher, A. H., Lynch, J. J., et al., "Animal companions and one-year survival of patients after discharge from a coronary care unit," *Public Health Reports 95* (1980): 307-12.

40 Seigel, J. M., "Stressful life events and use of physician services among the elderly: the moderating role of pet ownership," *Journal of Personality and Social Psychology 58* (1960): 1081-6.

41 Fawzy, F. I., Fawzy, N. W., Hyun, C. S., et al. Malignant melanoma effects of an early structured psychiatric intervention, coping and affective state on recurrence and survival 6 years later," *Arch Gen Psychiatry 50* (1993): 681-9).

42 Spiegel, D., Bloom, J. R., Kraemer, H. C., and E. Gottheil, "Effect of psychosocial treatment on survival of patients with metastatic breast cancer," *Lancet 2* (1989): 888-91.

43 Ornish, D., Brown, S. E., Scherwitz, L. W., et al., "Can lifestyle changes reverse coronary heart disease?" *Lancet 336* (1990): 129-33.

44 Ornish, D., Scherwitz, L., Billings, J., Gould, L., Sparler, T. S., Armstrong, W. T., Ports, T. A., Kirkeeide, R. L., Hogeboom, C., and R. Brand, "Intensive Lifestyle Changes for Reversal of Coronary Heart Disease," *JAMA 280* (1998): 2001-7.

45 Dr. Dean Ornish. *Love and Survival: The Scientific Basis for the Healing Power of Intimacy*, 2.

46 ibid., quote from p. 21.

47 Emoto, M., The True Power of Water: Healing and Discovering Ourselves (New York: Atria Books, 2003), 58-63.

48 Hay, L., *The Power is Within You* (Concord, NH: Specialist Publications), 19.

Chapter 6

1 Extracts from the Corpus Hippocraticum.

2 Vesalius, A., De Humanis Corporis Fabrica Libri Septum. Johannes Operinus, 1543.

THE EAGLE'S WAY

3   *Encyclopaedia Brittanica.*
4   *Concise Oxford Dictionary.*
5   ibid.
6   Extracts from the Corpus Hippocraticum.
7   The human genome project was completed in 2003 except for 8 percent, but work is ongoing.

Chapter 7

1   *Collins Australian Dictionary.*
2   R. F. C. Hull, trans., *The Collected Works of Carl G. Jung,* Bollingen Series XX (Princeton, NJ: Princeton University Press).
3   Sdorow L. Maslow's Hierarchy of Needs. Psychology, 327-328. Published by Wm. Brown, 1990.
4   Weiten W. Maslow's Theory of Self-Actualization. Psychology. Published by Brookes, Cole 1992; 442_443.
5   Grof, S., with Bennett, H. Z., *The Holotropic Mind: The Three Levels of Human Consciousness and How They Shape Our Lives* (New York: Harper, 1993).
6   Jung, C. G., *Memories, Dreams, Reflections* (New York: Vintage Press, 1989).
7   Lipton Bruce PhD. *The Biology of Belief.* Chapter One. *Lessons from the Petri dish. In praise of smart cells and smart students.* Hay House 2005
8   Tompkins, Peter, and Christopher Bird, *The Secret Life of Plants* (New York: HarperCollins, 1973).
9   Matthew's Gospel 7:7, Good News Bible.

Chapter 8

1   F. Capra, *The Tao of Physics* (New York: Flamingo, 1991), 149.
2   N. Bohr, *Atomic Physics and the Description of Nature* (London: Cambridge University Press, 1934), 57.
3   Capek, M., *The Philosophical Impact of Contemporary Physics* (Princeton, NJ: D Van Nostrand, 1961), 319.
4   Capra, F., *The Turning Point* (New York: HarperCollins, 1983), 76.
5   Schrodinger, E., *What is Life?* (New York: Macmillan, 1946), 145.
6   Capra, F., *The Turning Point* (New York: HarperCollins, 1983), 77

7 ibid., p. 85.

8 Platonov, K., *The Word as a Psychological and Therapeutic Factor* (Moscow: Foreign Language Publishing House, 1959).

9 Weatherhead, L. D., *Psychology, Religion and Healing* (Nashville: Abington Press, 1952).

10 Hurley, T. J. Multiple Personality—Mirrors of a New Model of Mind. Investigations 1. (Sausalito Calif): Institute of Noetic Sciences, 1985: 1-23.

11 *Encyclopaedia Brittanica*, 1999.

12 Eysenck, H. J., "Personality, stress and cancer: prediction and prophylaxis," *British Journal of Medical Psychology 61* (1988): 57-75.

13 Allison, T. G., Williams, D. E., Miller, D. E., et al., "Medical and economic costs of psychological distress in patients with coronary heart disease," *Mayo Clinic Proceedings 70* (1995): 734-42.

14 Mittelman, M. A., Maclure, M., Sherwood, J. B., et al., "Triggering of acute myocardial infarction onset by episodes of anger," Circulation 92 (1995): 1720-5.

15 Emoto, M., *The Power of Water: Healing and Discovering Ourselves* (New York: Atria Books, 2003), 13, 59, 62-3. Some of these photos can be viewed on his website at www.masaru-emoto.net/english/entop.html.

16 Springer, S. P., and Deutsch. 1999. Left brain, Right brain: Perspectives from Cognitive Neuroscience. NY. W. H. Freeman and Coy; 65

17 Norman Doidge, MD, *The Brain that Changes Itself. Revised Edition* (New York: Scribe Publications, 2008), 198.

18 Pascual-Leone, A., Nguyet, D., Cohen, L. G., Brasil-Neto, J. P., Cammarota, A., and M. Hallett, "Modulation of muscle responses evoked by transcranial magnetic stimulation during the acquisition of new fine motor skills, *J Neurophysiol 74* (1995): 1037-45.

19 Yue, G., and K. J. Cole, "Strength increases from the motor program: Comparison of training with maximal voluntary and imagined muscle contractions," Journal of Neurophysiology 67(5) (May 1992) 1114-23.

THE EAGLE'S WAY

20 Hochberg, L., Serruya, M. D., Friehs, G. M., Mukand, J. A., Saleh, M., Caplan A. H., Branner, A., Chen, D., Penn, R., and J. P. Donoghue, "Neuronal ensemble control of prosthetic devices by a human with tetraplegia," *Nature 442* (July 2006): 164-71.

21 Pert, C., *Molecules of Emotion: Why You Feel the Way You Do* (New York: Scribner, 1997).

22 ibid., p. 147.

23 ibid., p. 187.

24 Pearsall, P., *The Heart's Code: Tapping the Wisdom and Power of Our Heart Energy* (New York: Bantam Books, 1999), 4-8.

25 Pert, C., *Everything You Need To Feel Go(o)d* (Carlsbad, CA: Hay House, 2006. 53-4.

26 Sdorow, L., Humanistic Psychology: 464-6.

27 Frankl, V., *Man's Search for Meaning* (New York: Washington Square Press, 1959).

28 Talbot, M., *The Holographic Universe* (New York: HarperCollins, 1996).

29 ibid., from "Chapter Two: The Cosmos as Hologram."

30 Blake William. *Auguries of Innocence.*

Chapter 9

1 Magee, B., *The Story of Philosophy* (London: Dorling Kindersley, 2010).

2 Hawking, S., and L. Mlodinov, *The Grand Design* (New York: Bantam Books, 2010).

3 Richard Dawkins, *The God Delusion* (New York: Bantam Books, 2006).

4 Magee, B., *The Story of Philosophy* (London: Dorling Kindersley, 2010).

5 Wikipedia on Albert Einstein's life.

6 Albert Einstein, *Religion and Science.* New York Times. September 9, 1930.

7 Einstein Albert. Letter to Max Born December 4, 1926.

8 Dukas, H., and B. Hoffmann, Albert Einstein. The human sides: new glimpses from his archives. 1979

9   Chopra, D., and L. Mlodinow, *War of the Worldviews: Science v. Spirituality* (London: Rider Books, 2010), 298.

10   Ramana Maharshi, an Indian sage (1879-1950) introduced this way of self-enquiry. Paul Brunton wrote of this in *A Search in Secret India* (Rider & Co, 1931).

11   The King James Bible. Exodus 3:14.

12   ibid., Exodus 3:15.

13   ibid John 11:25.

14   ibid John 14:6.

15   Good News Bible, John 10:30.

16   ibid., John 14:10.

17   ibid., Luke 17: 21.

18   King James Bible, John 10:34.

19   ibid., Luke 11:2.

20   Ibid., John 1:9. 21

21   Quran 50:16.

22   Eckhart Tolle, *The Power of Now: A Guide to Spiritual Enlightenment.* (Hodder, 1999).

23   Eckhart Tolle, *A New Earth* (New York: Penguin, 2005).

24   Wikipedia

25   ibid.

26   ibid.

27   Lutz, A., Greischer, L., Rawlings, N., Ricard, M., and R. Davidson, "Long—. term meditators self-induced high-amplitude gamma synchrony during mental practice, *National Academy of Sciences of the United States of America 101* (November 16, 2004): 16, 369-73.

28   King James Bible. Matthew 16:25.

29   ibid., John 12:24-5.

30   Good News Bible. 1 Cor. 12:9-10.

31   ibid., Acts 5:12-16.

32   *Collins English Dictionary,* 2001.

33   Good News Bible, Matthew 13:10-17.

Chapter 10

1   This quote has been attributed to Bertrand Russell, but I have not been able to source it.

2   *Concise Oxford Dictionary.*

3   Aphorisms from the Corpus Hippocraticum.

4   Zwar, D., *Doctor Ahead of His Time: The Life of Psychiatrist Dr. Ainsley Meares* (Valencia, CA: Greenhouse Publications, 1985).

5   Grof, S., and C. Grof, *The Stormy Search for the Self: A Guide to Personal Growth through Transformational Crisis* (London: Mandala, HarperCollins, 1991).

6   Watkins, A., *Mind-Body Medicine: A Clinician's Guide to Psychoneuroimmunology* (London: Churchill Livingstone, 1997).

7   Ader, R., Felten, D., and N. Cohen, *Psychoneuroimmunology* (New York: Academic Press, 1991).

8   Eysenck, H. J., and R. Grossarth-Maticek, "Creative novation behaviour therapy as a prophylactic treatment for cancer and coronary heart disease: part 2—effects of treatment," *Behav Res Ther 29* (1991): 17-31.

9   Boris Pasternak won the Nobel Prize for literature in 1958 with Doctor Zhivago. Quote is from Vintage 2010 paperback edition (p. 432).

10   Bach, E., *Heal Thyself: An Explanation of the Real Cause and Cure of Disease* (London: CW Daniel Coy, Ltd., 1931).

11   Hay Louise, L., *You Can Heal Your Life* (Concord, NH: Specialist Publications, 1984).

12   In chronological order, the doctors who have written on medical metaphysics: Harrison, J., *Love Your Disease* (Angus & Robertson, 1984).
Dethlefsen and Dahlke, *The Healing Power of Illness* (Element Books, 1990).
Myss and Sheally, *The Creation of Health* (Stillpoint Publishing, 1993).
Schultz, M. L., *Awakening Intuition* (Harmony Books/Random House).

13   Myss, C., *Anatomy of the Spirit: The Seven Stages of Power and Healing* (New York: Harmony Books, 1996), 68.

DR. PETER L. JOHNSTON

14   Levine, S., "The Life of the Open Heart," from an interview with Eliot Jay Rosen in Sausalito, CA, in *Experiencing the Soul* (Hay House, 1998), 172.

Chapter 11

1   Matthew 11:13-15 and 17:11-13.
2   John: 9:2.
3   Wambach, H., *Life before Life* (New York: Bantam Books, 1984).
4   Weiss, B., *Many Lives, Many Masters* (New York: Simon & Schuster, 1988).
5   Schroder, T., *Old Souls: The Scientific Evidence for Past Lives* (1999).
6   Merzenich, M. M., Allard, T., W. M. and Jenkins, "Neural ontogeny of higher brain function. Implications of some recent neurophysiological findings" (1991).
7   R. F. C. Hull, trans., *The Collected Works of Carl G. Jung, Bollingen Series XX* (Princeton, NJ: Princeton University Press).
8   ibid.
9   Hal Stone and Sidra, *Embracing Our Selves: The Voice Dialogue Manual* (Nataraj Publishing, 1989).
10   Myss, C., and C. N. Shealy, *The Creation of Health: The Emotional, Psychological and Spiritual Responses that Promote Health and Healing* (New York: Bantam Books, 1998).
11   Herbert Benson MD with Miriam Z.Klipper. *The Relaxation Response.* Collins 1975.

Chapter 12

1   Grof, S., *The Transpersonal Vision: The Healing Potential of Non-Ordinary States of Consciousness* (Boulder, CO: Sounds True, 1998). Weiss, B., *Many Lives, Many Masters* (New York: Simon & Schuster, 1988).
2   St. John of the Cross (1542-1591). "Dark Night of the Soul" from the *Collected Works of Saint John of the Cross.* ICS publications.
3   Grof, S., and C. Grof, *The Stormy Search for the Self: Understanding and Living with Spiritual Emergency* (London: Mandala HarperCollins, 1991), 56-7.

THE EAGLE'S WAY

4   O'Connor, P., *Understanding the Mid-life Crisis* (Sun, Australia: 1981).

5   Lynch, J. J., *The Broken Heart: The Medical Consequences of Loneliness* (New York: Basic Books, 1977).

6   Stone, H., and S. L. Stone, *Embracing Each Other: Relationship as Teacher, Healer and Guide* (Nataraj Publishing, 1989).

7   Hendrix, H., *Getting the Love You Want: A Guide for Couples* (Schwartz & Wilkinson, 1998).

8   Dossey, L., *Healing Words: The Power of Prayer and the Practice of Medicine* (New York: Harper Collins, 1993).

9   Rob Brezsny, *Pronoia Is the Antidote for Paranoia* (San Rafael, CA: Frog, Ltd., and Televisionary Publishing, 2005).

Chapter 13

1   Le Fanu.

2   Witschi, H., "A short history of lung cancer," *Toxicological Sciences 64:1* (November 2001): 4-6.

3   "Interview with Sir Richard Doll," originally published in *Icon Issue 1* (2005).

4   National Institutes of Health (April 10, 1998), Background on cigar monograph: Cigars: health effects and trends.

5   Kuper, H., Bofetta, P., and H. Adami, "Tobacco use and cancer causation: Association by tumour type," *Journal of Internal Medicine 252: 3* (2002): 206-24.

6   Lipworth, L., Tarone, R., and J. McLaughlin, "The Epidemiology of Renal Cell Carcinoma," *The Journal of Urology 176: 6* (2006): 2353-8.

7   Iodice, S., Gandini, S., Maisonneuve, P., and A. B. Lowenfels, "Tobacco and the risk of pancreatic cancer: A review and meta-analysis," *Langenbeck's Archives of Surgery 393: 4* (2008): 535.

8   Bofetta, P., "Tobacco smoking and risk of bladder cancer, *Scandinavian Journal of Urology and Nephrology 42* (2002): 45-54.

9   Cui, Y., Miller, A., and T. Rohan, "Cigarette smoking and breast cancer risk: Update of a prospective cohort study," *Breast Cancer Research and Treatment 100: 3* (2006): 293-9.

10 Calle, E., Miracle-McMahill, H., Thun, M. J., and C. W. Heath, Jr., "Cigarette smoking and risk of fatal breast cancer," American Journal of Epidemiology. 139 (10):1001-7

11 Bonita, R., Scragg, R., Stewart, A., et al., "Cigarette smoking and risk of premature stroke in men and women," *British Medical Journal Clinical Research Ed. 293* (1986): 6-8

12 Shinton, R., and G. Beevers, "Meta-analysis of relation between cigarette smoking and stroke," *British Medical Journal 298* (1989): 789-94

13 Alexander, R., Diabetes Dialectics: Statistics from the Independent (2011).

14 Le Fanu.

15 Le Fanu reference to Doll.

16 Burkitt Denis. Bio on Wikipedia.

17 "American Journal of Clinical Nutrition," last visited on January 13, 2010.

18 Dr. Mehmet, *TIME Magazine*, September 12, 2011.

19 Harvard School of Public Health 2005. 12,829 children aged nine to fourteen. Weight gain with skim and 1 percent milk but not with dairy fat milk.

20 Cancer Res 35: 3513. 1975

21 Koh, L., "An Asian perspective to the problem of osteoporosis," *Ann Acad Med Singapore 31* (January 2002): 26-9.

22 Alexander, R., Diabetes Dialectics (2011).

23 Durazo-Arvizu, R., McGee, D., Cooper, R., Liao, R., and A. Luke, "Mortality and optimal body mass index in a sample of the US population," American Journal of Epidemiology 147 (1998): 739-49.

24 McGee, D. L., "Body mass index and mortality: A meta-analysis based on personal-level data from twenty-six observational studies," *Ann Epidemiology 15* (2005): 87-97.

25 Flegal, K., Graubard, B., Williamson, D., and M. Gail, "Supplement: Response to "'Can Fat Be Fit?'" *Scientific American 297* (2008): 5-6.

26 Janssen, I., and A. E. Mark, "Elevated body mass index and mortality risk in the elderly," *Obesity Review 8* (2007): 41-59.

THE EAGLE'S WAY

27　Ross, C., Langer R. D., and E. Barrett-Connor, "Given diabetes, is it fat better than thin?" *Diabetes Care 20* (1997): 650-2.

28　Barrett-Connor, E., and K. Khaw, "Is hypertension more benign when associated with obesity?" Circulation 72 (1985): 53_60.

29　Morse, S., Gulati, R., and E. Riesin, "The obesity paradox and cardiovascular disease," *Curr Hypertens Rep 12* (2010): 120-6.

30　Barrett-Connor, E., "Obesity, atherosclerosis and coronary artery disease." *Ann Internal Medicine 103* (1985): 1010-19.

31　Kang, X., Shaw, L. J., Hayes, S., Hachamovitch, R., Abidov, A., Cohen, I., Friedman, J., Thomson, L., Polk, D., Germano, D., and D. Berman, "Impact of body mass index on cardiac mortality in patients with known or suspected coronary artery disease undergoing myocardial perfusion single-photon emission computed tomography," *Journal American College of Cardiology 47* (2006): 1418-26.

32　Beddhu, S., "The body mass index paradox and an obesity, inflammation and atherosclerosis syndrome in chronic kidney disease," *Seminars in Dialysis 17* (2004): 229-32.

33　Kulminski, A., Arbeev, K., Kulminskaya, I., Ukraintseva, S., Land, K., Akusevich, I., and A. Yashin, "Body mass index and nine-year mortality in disabled and nondisabled older US individuals," *Journal American Geriatric Society 56* (2008): 105-10.

34　Dr R. Kausman, "If not dieting then what?" *Allen and Unwin* (1998): 5

35　Mann, T., Tomiyama, A., Westling, E., Lew, A., Samuels, B., Chatman, J., "Medicare's Search for Effective Obesity Treatments: Diets are not the answer," *Am Psychol 62* (2007): 220-33.

36　Howard, B., Manson, J., Stefanick, M., Beresford, S., Frank, G., Jones, B., Rodabough, R., Snetselaar, L., Thomson, C., Tinker, L., et al., "Low fat dietary pattern and weight change over seven years: The Women's Health Initiative Dietary Modification Trial," JAMA 295 (2006): 39-49.

37　National Institutes of Health (NIH), "Methods for voluntary weight loss and control (Technology Assessment Conference Panel)," *Ann Internal Medicine 116* (1992): 942-9.

38 Ingram, D., and M. Mussolino, "Weight loss from maximum body weight and mortality: The Third National Health and Nutrition Examination Survey Linked Mortality File," *International Journal Obesity 24* (2010): 1044-50.

39 Bacon, L., Stern, J., Keim, N., and M. Van Loan, "Low bone mass in premenopausal chronic dieting obese women." *Eur J Clin Nutrition 58* (2004): 966-71.

40 Barr, S., Prior, J., and Y Vigna, "Restrained eating and ovulatory disturbances. Possible implications for bone health," *Am J Clin Nutrition 59* (1994): 92-7.

41 Van Loan, M., Bachrach, I., Wang, M., and P. Crawford, "Effect of drive for thinness during adolescence on adult bone mass," *J Bone Mineral Res 15* (2000): 5412.

42 Chevrier, J., Dewally, E., Ayotte, P., Mauriege, P., Despres, J., and A. Tremblay, "Body weight loss increases plasma and adipose tissue concentrations of potentially toxic pollutants in obese individuals," *Int J Obesity Relat Metab Disorders 24* (2000): 1272-8.

43 Puhl, R., Andreyeva, T., and K. Brownell, "Perceptions of weight discrimination; prevalence and comparison to race and gender discrimination in America," *Int Journal Obesity 32* (2008): 992-1000.

44 Haines, J., Neumark-Sztainer, D., and M. Eisenberg, "Weight teasing and disordered eating behaviour in adolescents: Longtitudinal findings from project EAT (Eating Among Teens)," *Paediatrics 117* (2006): e209-15.

45 Storch, E., Milsom, V., Debraganza, N., Lewin, A., Geffken, G., and J. Silverstein, "Peer victimization, psychosocial adjustment and physical activity in overweight and at-risk-for-overweight youth," *Journal of Paediatric Psychology 32* (2007): 80-89.

46 Vartanian, I., and J. Shaprow, "Effects of weight stigma on exercise motivation and behaviour: A preliminary investigation among college-aged females," *J of Health Psychol 13* (2008): 131-8.

47 Puhl, R., and C. Heuer, "The stigma of obesity: A review and update," Obesity 17 (2009): 941-64.

THE EAGLE'S WAY

48 Amy, N., Aalborg, A., Lyons, P., and L. Keranen, "Barriers to routine gynaecological cancer screening for white and African-American obese women," *Int J Obes Relat Metab Disord 30* (2006): 147-55.

49 Faith, M., Leone, M., Ayers, T., Heo, M., and A. Pietrobelli, "Weight criticism during physical activity, coping skills and reported physical activity in children," *Paediatrics 110* (2002): e23.

50 Dr. R. Kausman, "If not dieting then what?" *Allen and Unwin* (1998).

51 Linda Bacon PhD. *Health at every Size.* Kindle edition.

52 Adapted from Dr. Rick Kausman's book *If Not Dieting, then What?* (p. 199-202).

Chapter 14

1 Moody, R., *Life After Life: The 25th Anniversary Edition* (Ryder, 2001).

2 Filmed interview with Dr. Moody in Chicago, described by J. R. Rosen in his collected interviews *Experiencing the Soul* (87-8).

3 Filmed interview with Prof. K. J. Ring in Connecticut by Eliot Jay Rosen in his collected interviews *Experiencing the Soul* (238).

4 ibid., p. 242.

5 Rosen, E. J., Interview with Elisabeth Kubler-Ross at her home in Arizona in *Experiencing the Soul* (5-13).

6 ibid., interview with Dr. Moody (88).

7 ibid., interview with Kenneth Ring, PhD (240).

8 Near-death experiences and the After Life website: neardeath.com

9 ibid., interview with Bill Guggenheim by Eliot Rosen in Arizona (61-71).

10 ibid.

11 Osis, K., and E. Haraldsson, *Deathbed Observations by Physicians and Nurses* (Parapsychology Foundation, 1961).

12 Bill and Judy Guggenheim, *After-Death Communication: Joyous Reunions with Deceased Loved Ones* (http://www.after death. com/about/adc.htm).

13 Goleman, D., *Emotional Intelligence: Why It Can Matter More than IQ* (Bloomsbury, 1996).

14 Childre, D., and H. Martin, *The Heartmath Solution* (San Francisco: HarperSanFrancisco, 1999), 9.

15 Armour, J., and J. Ardell, *Neurocardiology* (New York: Oxford University Press, 1984).

16 LeDoux, J., *The Emotional Brain: The Mysterious Underpinnings of Emotional Life* (New York: Simon and Schuster, 1996).

17 Childre, D., and H. Martin, *The Heartmath Solution* (San Francisco: Harper, 1999), 9.

18 ibid.

19 Lacey, J., and B. Lacey, "Some autonomic-central nervous system interrelationships." In Black P, Physiological Correlates of Emotion. New York: Academic Press, 1970: 205_227.

20 ibid.

21 Cantin, M., and J. Genest, "The Heart as an Endocrine Gland," Scientific American 254:2 (1986): 76-81.

22 Song, L., Schwartz, G., and L. Russek, "Heart-focused attention and heart-brain synchronization: Energetic and physiological mechanisms," *Alternative Therapies in Health and Medicine* 4:5 (1998): 44-52.

23 Grof, S., *The Transpersonal Vision* (Tapes by Sounds True, 1998).

24 Bays, B., *The Journey* (London: HarperCollins, 1999).

25 De Castella, N., Keys to Emotional Mastery: A personal discussion with author (1998).

26 Walsch, N. D., *What God Wants* (Hodder Mobius, 2005), 156-7.

Chapter 15

1 A Course in Miracles © 1975, 1992. Foundation for a Course in Miracles. Temelua: 1985.

2 Jampolsky, J., *Out of Darkness into the Light: A Journey of Inner Healing*, (Bantam Books, 1989), 79.

3 Although there were many, some I still have in my library are: Bailes, F., *Your Mind Can Heal You* (De Vorss & Co., 1941). Goldsmith, J., *Practising the Presence* (Fowler & Co., 1956). Macdonald-Bayne, M., *Divine Healing of Mind and Body* (Fowler & Co., 1953).

4   Walsch, N. D., *Conversations with God: Australia and New Zealand Edition* (Hodder and Stoughton, 1996).

5   *Concise Oxford Dictionary.*

6   Pert, C., *Molecules of Emotion: Why You Feel the Way You Do* (New York: Scribner,1997).

7   For a recent update on these metaphysical principles, I recommend this book: E. and J. Hicks, *Ask and It Is Given: Learning to Manifest Your Desires* (Hay House, 2004).

8   Benor, D., *Healing Research: Vol. 1* (Holistic Healing Publications).

9   Dean, E. D., High-Voltage Radiation Photography of a Healer's Finger. From The Kirlian Aura: Photographing the Galaxies of Life. eds. Stanley Krippner and Daniel Rubin (New York: Anchor Books, 1974).

10 Emoto, M., *Love Thyself: The Message from Water: Book 3* (Hay House, 2006), X111-x1x.

11 Levine, S., *Who Dies: An Investigation of Conscious Living and Conscious Dying* (Bath: Gateway Books, 1986).

12 Dossey, L., *Energy Medicine: Subtle Energies, Consciousness and the New Science of Healing* (Sounds True, 1998).

Chapter 16

1   Becker, R., *Cross Currents: The Perils of Electropollution. The Promise of Electromedicine* (New York: Tarcher/Penguin, 1990), 41-2.

2   Sheldrake, R., *A New Science of Life* (1981).

3   Pert, C., PhD, Everything You Need to Feel Go(o)d (Hay House, 2007)

4   Veith, I., *The Yellow Emperor's Classic of Internal Medicine* (University of California Press, 1949).

Chapter 17

1   Butler-Bowdon, T., *50 Psychology Classics* (Nicholas Brearley Publishing, 2007), 114.

2   Ibid., p. 270.

3   Covey, S., *The 8th Habit: From Effectiveness to Greatness* (Free Press, 2005), 43.

DR. PETER L. JOHNSTON

4 Norman Doidge, MD, *The Brain that Changes Itself: Revised Edition* (New York: Scribe Publications, 2008), 199-200.

5 Pascual-Leone, A., and F. Torres, "Plasticity of the sensorimotor cortex representation of the reading finger in Braille readers," *Brain 116* (1993): 39-52.

6 Pascual-Leone, A., Hamilton, R., Tormos, J., Keenan, J., and M. Catala, (1999): 94-108.

7 Norman Doidge, MD, *The Brain that Changes Itself: Revised Edition* (New York: Scribe Publications, 2008), 59.

8 Norman Doidge, MD. *The Brain that Changes Itself: Revised Edition* (New York: Scribe Publications, 2008), 59-60.

9 Gage, F., Van Praag, H., Schinder, A., Christie, B., Toni, N., and T. Palmer, "Neurogenesis in the adult hippocampus," *Nature Medicine 4:11* (1998): 1313-7.

10 Van Praag, H., Kempermann, G., and F. Gage, "Running increases cell proliferation and neurogenesis in the adult mouse dentate gyrus," *Nature Neuroscience 2* (1999): 266-70.

11 Wilson, R., Mendes de Leon, C., Barnes, L., Schneider, J., Bienias, J., Evans, D., and D. Bennett, "Participation in cognitively stimulating activities and risk of incident Alzheimer Disease," *JAMA 287:6* (2002):742-8.

12 Lauren, D., Verreault, R., Lindsay, J., MacPherson, K., and K. Rockwood, "Physical activity and risk of cognitive impairment and dementia in elderly persons," *Arch Neurol 58* (March 2001).

13 Kempermann, G., Gast, D., and F. Gage, "Neuroplasticity in old age: Sustained fivefold induction of hippocampal neurogenesis by long-term environmental enrichment," *Annals of Neurology 52* (2002): 135-43.

14 Verghese, J., Lipton, R., Katz, M., Hall, C., Derby, C., Kuslansky, G., Ambrose, A., Sliwinski, M., and H. Buschke, "Leisure activities and the risk of dementia in the elderly," *New England Journal of Medicine 348: 25* (2003): 2508-16.

15 Vaillant, G., *Aging Well: Surprising Guideposts to a Happier Life from the Landmark Harvard Study of Adult Development* (Boston: Little Brown & Co., 2002).

16 Lehman, H., *Age and Achievement* (Princeton, NJ: Princeton University Press, 1953). Simonton, D., "Does creativity decline in the later years?" *Definition, data and theory* (1990). M. Permutter, *Late Life Potential* (Washington, DC: Gerontologial Soc of America), 83-112.
17 Gardner, H., *Frames of Mind* (New York: Basic Books, 1985).
18 Tenosynovitis and De Quervains tenovaginitis are the medical terms for these afflictions.
19 WHO. Men, Aging and Health. Achieving Health across the Life Span. WHO Geneva 1999, 10.
20 Weiten, W., *Psychology: Themes and Variations* (Brooks Cole, 1992), 443-4.
21 Sdorow. Psychology. Wm C Brown Publishers Iowa 1990. Pge 463. Quoted from
22 Maslow, A. H., *The Farther Reaches of Human Nature* (New York: Viking Press, 1971).
23 Ibid.
24 Wikipedia

Chapter 18
1 *Concise Oxford Dictionary*
2 Childre, D., and H. Martin, *The Heartmath Solution* (San Francisco: Harper, 1999), 9.
3 Lee, A., and M. L. Done, "Stimulation of the wrist acupuncture point P6 for preventing postoperative nausea and vomiting," *Cochrane Database of Systemic Reviews 3* (2004).
4 Melchart, D., Linde, K., Berman, B., White, A., Vickers, A., Allies, G., and B. Brinkhaus, "Acupuncture for idiopathic headache," Cochrane Database of Systemic Reviews 1 (2001).
5 Benor, D., *Healing Research: Vol. 1* (Holistic Healing Publications).

Chapter 19
1 Mowrey, D., Herbal Tonic Remedies (Keats Publications, 1993). This book lists many clinical trials on herbs.

DR. PETER L. JOHNSTON

2   Linde, K., Clausius, N., Ramirez, G., et al., "Are the clinical effects of homeopathy placebo effects? A meta-analysis of place-bo-controlled trials," *Lancet 350* (1997): 834-43.

3   Kneijnen, J., Knipschild, P., and G. Ter Riet, "Clinical trials of homeopathy," *BMJ 302* (1991): 316-23.

4   Pomeranz, B., "Scientific Research into Acupuncture for the relief of pain," *The Journal of Alternative and Complementary Medicine 2:1* (1996): 53-60.

5   Flocco, B., "PMS Reflexology Research Study," Journal of Obstetrics and Gynaecology 82: 6 (December 1993).

6   AHMA website, *http://holisticmedicine.org/About.htm.*

7   Gibran, Kahlil. *The Prophet*, originally published in 1926. My quote from paperback edition (Pan Books, 1983), 612.

8   O'Regan, B., and C. Hirschberg, *Spontaneous Remission: An Annotated Bibliography* (Sausalito, CA: Institute of Noetic Sciences, 1993).

9   Quotation from Hippocrates Epidemics VI, Ch. 5, translated by W. H. S. Jones. and quoted by D. S. Sobel, ed. from the *Works of Hippocrates in Ways of Health* (New York: Harcourt Brace, 1979), 194. I obtained this quote from *Heart of Healing.* (Institute of Noetic Sciences, 1993)

10   *Concise Oxford Dictionary*

11   Encyclopaedia Brittanica 1999

12   ibid.

Chapter 20

1   WHO joint mission report Feb 28: *Mortality Rate in China as of February 2020.*

2   Ibid

3   Centers for Disease Control and Protection (CDC): *1918 Pandemic (H1N1 virus)*

4   Unfortunately, I cannot recall the sources but we are seeing spontaneous cases of COVID-19 appearing with no known connection to known cases. Also health personnel are continuing to work with inadequate protective equipment and not all of them are succumbing to infection.

THE EAGLE'S WAY

5   Video – *Chinese Medical Workers on the front line of the Coronavirus fight in Wuhan.* February 20th 2020.

6   Philippians 4:7 7

7   John 17:16

8   N.D.Walsch. *Conversations With God. Book 1. Australia and New Zealand edition.* Hodder and Stoughton 1996.

9   Christina Nunez. *Climate 101. Deforestation.* National Geographic. Feb 2019

10 Rich Gilmore. Director of the Nature Conservancy in Australia: *Australia's Bushfire Crisis.* Feb 12th 2020.

11 John Mecklin, editor. *2020 Doomsday Clock Statement of Scientific & Security Board of the Atomic Scientists.*

12 Jonathan Watts and Niko Commenda: *Coronavirus pandemic leading to huge drop in air pollution.* The Guardian 23rd March 2020

13 Renewable Resources Coalition: *Overpopulation: The Causes, Effects and Potential Solutions.* Based on UN figures 2016

GLOSSARY OF THERAPIES

Acupuncture: CAM in which fine needles are inserted in the skin at specific points along meridians. Meridians in TCM are fourteen energy lines traversing the body that are invisible to the naked eye.

Aerobic exercise regimes: Physical exercises focusing on improving the efficiency of the cardiovascular system in absorbing and transporting oxygen.

Affirmations: Statements of positive intent. Used to overcome habitual negative beliefs, they are stated in present tense and used regularly for this purpose.

Alexander technique: CAM designed to promote well-being by retraining one's awareness and habits of posture to ensure minimal effort and strain.

Angel cards: Divination systems based on spiritual messengers. There are at least five different decks of cards available for this purpose.

Anthroposophy: A system established by the Austrian philosopher Rudolf Steiner for optimising health and well-being.

Archetypal cards: A series of cards depicting archetypes. Carolyn Myss devised this system to be used in combination with astrological houses. The resultant chart helps clients in gaining psychological insights.

Aromatherapy: CAM using essential oils and aromatic plant extracts for therapeutic purposes.

THE EAGLE'S WAY

Art therapy: The use of art, sketching, and clay modelling as a means of accessing deeper issues.

Astrology: The study of celestial bodies, their positions, and their movements relative to Earth and time, together with the influences these have on individual and collective human attitudes and behaviours.

Ayervedic medicine: A holistic, comprehensive system of health care derived from India. Its origins go back five thousand years.

Behavioural therapy (behaviourism): The theory that human behaviour can be explained in terms of conditioning and that psychological disorders are best treated by altering behaviour patterns.

Bio-electronic devices: CAM devices measuring bio-energies. Starting with Voll's Dermatron, there are now quite a number of more sophisticated machines: Vega, Mora, and Listen, to name a few. They are useful in measuring food and drug intolerances, vitamin and mineral deficiencies, and biological age. Mora and Listen machines can recommend homeopathic remedies and even manufacture them electronically.

Bioenergetics: CAM based on the work of Wilhelm Reich, a student of Sigmund Freud. Bioenergetics theory postulates that emotional healing can be aided by resolving body tension. Postures and exercises are central to this.

Biofeedback: Electronic monitoring of a normally automatic body function in order to train a person to acquire some voluntary control over that function.

Bio-identical hormones: Hormones identical to those in the body. Although yet unproven in trials, the movement toward these has arisen from a perception that synthetic hormones, especially progestogens, produce greater side effects than natural hormones.

Body dialogue: A counselling technique using a gestalt process on organs or body systems in order to access inner wisdom.

Bowen therapy: CAM originated by Tom Bowen and using relatively gentle manipulation of muscles to release energy, thereby aiding self-healing.

CAM: Complementary/alternative medical treatment.

331

DR. PETER L. JOHNSTON

Chakra balancing: In the Indian system, chakras are vortices of energy acting as reservoirs of energy and information and as valves allowing appropriate amounts of energy to flow in and out of the physical body. Balancing the chakras is a CAM, which focuses on balancing the seven main chakras that are located in the head and trunk.

Channelling: Known also as "mediumship." People who can transmit information from other dimensions are called "channels." Most psychics do this while fully conscious. Others are "trance channels" allowing their bodies to be used by angels or evolved, disembodied beings for the transmission of information to others.

Chelation: In medicine, the use of a chemical called EDTA as a detoxification method in heavy metal poisoning. In CAM, especially nutritional medicine, chelation is used to reduce the cholesterol levels in patients with established heart disease.

Chemotherapy: Treatment of disease, mainly cancer, by chemical means.

Chinese astrology: Like European astrology, it relates birthdate with character traits, but the Chinese system focuses on the year of birth rather than the day.

Chiropractic: CAM based on diagnosis and manipulative treatment of misalignment in the spinal column and joints.

Clinical ecology: CAM with special interest in the effects on the body of chemicals, additives, and pollutants in food, water, and air.

Cognitive behavioural therapy: A psychotherapeutic approach wherein dysfunctional patterns of thought—about one's self and one's world—are challenged.

Colour therapy: CAM in which colours are used to enhance healing. **Computerised axial tomography (CT scanning):** Fine X-ray beams applied in a rotary fashion to produce an image of the body or body parts in cross sections.

Conventional Western medicine (or orthodox medicine or mainstream medicine): Medical practice conforming to generally accepted beliefs and practices. The way it is usually done.

THE EAGLE'S WAY

Cupping: Ancient Chinese practice in which suction cups are applied over areas of pain and acupuncture points. Used in lung and bowel conditions as well as the relief of pain.

Cranial osteopathy: CAM focusing on gentle palpation and visualisation of the skull bones. Because the practitioner tunes in to a subtle bio-energetic pulsation, the therapy belongs to bio-energetic rather than physical medicine.

Crystals: In the same way they were used in early radios, crystals are used to amplify healing in pranic or spiritual healing. Coloured crystals of various types are also used to aid emotional states and spiritual growth.

Cutting the ties that bind: Founded by Phyllis Crystal as a way of providing an inner puberty rite for Westerners, it has been expanded to help people move on from constricting relationships and phobias. It combines aspects of bio-energetic medicine as well as counselling and can be a powerful source of insights.

Diathermy of cervix: A conventional medical procedure in which premalignant conditions of the uterine cervix are ablated (burned off).

Divination systems: Divination is defined as the practice of seeking knowledge by supernatural means. With holism now being recognised as applying to matter and consciousness, divination may not be as supernatural as originally thought.

Dowsing: Defined as water divining. In CAM, rods or pendulums can be used as an aid to making choices in a wide range of issues concerning health.

Dream interpretation: Described by Freud and Jung as the "royal road to the unconscious," it is still a very useful counselling technique for accessing insights.

Dreamtime: In Aboriginal legend, Dreamtime or *Alcheringa* is the golden age when the first ancestors were created.

Ear candling: Technique used by ancient Egyptians, Chinese, and Hopi Indians. Hollow candle lit and used to extract old wax and fungus. Claims made for stimulating the immune system.

Electro-acupuncture: Acupuncture using electrodes connected to the needles.

Electrocardiograph (ECG): Medical device that measures the bio-electric activity of the heart.

Electroencephalograph (EEG): Medical device that measures the electrical activity of the brain—the so-called brain waves.

Electrotherapy: Devices using electric impulses in healing. The most widely used is the TENS machine in pain management.

Endoscopy: Medical procedure used for viewing the internal structure of hollow organs (e.g., stomach, bowel, bladder, and uterus).

Enneagram: An ancient system that classifies people into nine categories. Each category is further divided into nine levels ranging from highly evolved down to psychologically disturbed. With eighty-one archetypes, it is a remarkably comprehensive system that can provide insights for the seeker.

Exclusion diets: Diets excluding foods to which an individual shows intolerance.

Eye movement desensitisation and reprocessing (EMDR): Psychotherapy useful in treating stress and phobias. Moving the eyes from side to side while visualising a stressful episode appears to bring the left and right hemispheres of the brain into balance. This allows resolution of the emotional reactivity to the stress.

Feldenkrais method: CAM designed to promote physical and mental well-being by analysis of neuromuscular activity. It employs exercises that improve flexibility and coordination.

Flower essences: Essences derived from flowers at their peak of bloom, used as an aid to the healing of emotional and mental states. Pioneered by Dr. Edward Bach in the 1920s, essences are now found globally. Pacific Essences and Australian Bush Flower Essences are popular here in Australia.

Food sensitivity testing: IgG-mediated allergies to foods can be detected by using blood tests. Such life-threatening allergies are fortunately uncommon. More frequently, people are intolerant rather than allergic to foods. Confirming the diagnosis of intolerance is not as easy. Techniques for food testing include pulse

THE EAGLE'S WAY

testing, exclusion and challenge, bio-electronic devices, and kinesiology. None are 100 per cent accurate, but all are useful.

Gem essences: Essences using energy of crystals.

Gestalt therapy: Role-playing technique in which one imagines one's self as a person, an animal, or a symbol for the purpose of gaining insights.

Group therapy: A form of psychiatric therapy in which patients meet to discuss their problems, usually mediated by a psychiatrist.

Hair analysis: The most accurate system currently available for measuring heavy metal toxicity. Also useful for assessing body mineral levels.

Hakomi: A psychotherapeutic system especially useful for psychological trauma.

Herbalism: The study or practice of the medicinal and therapeutic use of plants.

History taking: Clarifying a client's problem by taking details of the presenting problem and asking questions relative to the problem and the client's life.

Holistic medicine: Treatment aimed at the whole person—body, mind, emotions, and spirit.

Holotropic breathwork: Psychotherapy in an altered state of consciousness induced by circular breathing, playing music, and sometimes touching.

Homeopathy: CAM in which disease is treated by minute doses of natural substances that in a healthy person would produce symptoms similar to those of the presenting disease. Founded by Dr. Samuel Hahnemann in the late eighteenth century, it went into decline with the arrival of antibiotics in mid-twentieth century but is now undergoing a renaissance.

Humanistic psychology: Founded by Maslow and Rogers in the 1950s as a counter to the behavioural and psychoanalytic perspectives, both of which saw humanity as victims—one to environmental stimuli, the other to unconscious motives. The focus of humanistic psychology is the individual's unique experience of the world.

Hypnotherapy: The use of hypnosis in therapy.

335

I Ching: An ancient Chinese manual of divination based on eight symbolic trigrams and sixty-four hexagrams interpreted in terms of the polarities of yin and yang.

Imago relationship therapy: Counselling technique introduced by Harville Hendrix for couples. Imago is an idealised but usually unconscious image of someone that influences a person's behaviour. Imago therapy focuses on facilitating partners to see each other fully and honestly.

Inner child cards: Tarot cards translated into fairy-tale images. They can be used to gain insights in a somewhat less confronting way than the standard tarot deck.

Inner child work: Psychotherapy focused on the inner child—the archetype that never grows old and dwells within every human being.

Integrative medicine: Similar to holistic medicine in treating the whole person. It mainly applies to medical practitioners integrating mainstream and holistic medicines.

Intestinal permeability testing: Testing for malabsorption. This testing is more a CAM procedure to confirm Candida overgrowth in the bowel, as conventional medicine does not recognise candidiasis as a cause of malabsorption.

Intuitive diagnosis: Diagnosis of energy dysfunctions in the body using intuition only. Intuition implies the ability to understand something immediately without using conscious reasoning. Intuitive readings can provide medical diagnoses and metaphysical causes in addition to the bio-energetic dysfunctions.

Iridology: CAM using the iris as an aid to diagnosis. Most naturopaths use the system founded by Von Peczely in the nineteenth century. It helps assess the nutritional state of organs and gives some guidance to stress levels.

Journaling: The practice of writing about one's goals and emotions. Regular practice brings insights and discipline toward one's intentions and overall life purpose.

Journeywork: A technique developed by Brandon Bays that helped her spontaneously resolve a basketball-sized tumour in the pelvis. It utilises a number of CAM psychotherapies, includ-

THE EAGLE'S WAY

ing visualisation, forgiveness, cutting ties, loving one's disease, NLP, and going through the emotional layers to find the love underneath.

Kabbalah: An ancient Jewish mystical tradition sometimes called "the Tree of Life."

Kinesiology: Defined as the study of the mechanics of body movements, it holds an important place in physiotherapy. In CAM, muscle strength can be used as a diagnostic indicator for a whole range of conditions, physical, mental, and environmental.

Kirlian photography: A technique for recording images of coronal discharges and the auras of living creatures.

Laser acupuncture: The use of laser beams instead of needles in acupuncture.

Lifeline technique: Uses kinesiology to access the subconscious and the mantra of love and gratitude to help transform underlying emotional and energetic patterns affecting health.

Live blood analysis: uses dark field microscopy of live blood to diagnose nutritional deficiencies and yeast overgrowth.

Logotherapy: A form of humanistic psychology initiated by Dr. Victor Frankl that focuses on life purpose.

Luscher colour therapy: Psychotherapy centred around the selection of eight or sixty-four colours.

Macrobiotics: A dietary system of whole foods prepared according to principles of yin/yang balance.

Magnet therapy: The use of magnets applied to the skin for the relief of pain in musculoskeletal problems.

Magnetic resonance imaging (MRI): A medical diagnostic procedure that makes use of strong magnetic fields and radiofrequency pulses to generate sectional images of the body in any plane.

Mainstream: Normal or conventional ideas, attitudes, or activities.

Massage: A kneading of muscles and joints to relieve tension or pain.

Medicine cards: Devised by Sams and Carson, the cards are based on the medicine wheel of Native-American culture.

Meditation: The practice of focusing the mind. Observing thoughts and detaching from them, when practised over the long term, gives the meditator a measure of control over an otherwise busy mind. It also helps the meditator to know the immortal Self.

Meridian-based psychotherapies: Psychotherapies in which individuals apply pressure to acupuncture points while the patients focus on their issues.

Mindfulness-based cognitive therapy: psychotherapy based on Jon Kabat-Zinn's mindfulness techniques for reducing stress. It has been shown to give help to patients with depression.

Modality: A method or procedure.

Music therapy: The use of music, toning, and harmonic sound for purposes of healing.

Natural vision methods: Exercises and techniques to improve ocular muscles, thereby improving vision without resorting to spectacles and contact lenses.

Network chiropractic: A system of diagnosis and treatment involving light touch rather than manipulation. It aims at emotional release and energy-based healing.

Neuro-linguistic programming (NLP): Psychotherapeutic system involving the linking of experiences with physical sensations.

Neuro-structural therapy: An extension of Bowen therapy involving energy release.

Nuclear scanning: The use of nuclear isotopes to image specific body systems (e.g., bone scans and PET scans).

Numerology: The branch of knowledge concerned with the esoteric significance of numbers.

Nutritional medicine: CAM focused on the role of nutrition and assimilation in health and disease. Many of its practitioners are medically trained doctors.

Orthomolecular psychiatry: CAM with special interest in nutritional aspects of mental health.

Osteopathy: CAM treating medical disorders through manipulation and massage of the skeleton and musculature.

Palmistry: The art or practice of interpreting people's characters or predicting their futures by examining their hands.

THE EAGLE'S WAY

Papanicolou smears: Better known as pap smears, where cells are taken from the uterine cervix to test for malignant and premalignant conditions.

Pathology testing: In medicine, using body tissues and body fluids to detect disease.

Pharmaceutical medicines: Medications or drugs produced by pharmaceutical companies. They account for almost all medical prescriptions.

Physical examination: Examining the physical body, whether still or in motion.

Physiotherapy: The treatment of disease, injury, or deformity by physical methods like massage and exercise rather than by drugs or surgery.

Pilates: A system for physical fitness with special emphasis on coordinating mind, body, and breath. It originated in World War I as a rehab system for returning veterans.

Postural integration: A form of deep tissue massage aimed at helping correct chronic dysfunctional postures.

Pranic healing: A form of spiritual healing based on Eastern energy anatomy.

Primal therapy: Psychotherapy introduced by Janov to access primitive emotions.

Psychoanalysis: Psychotherapy aiming to bring repressed fears and conflicts into consciousness where hopefully they can be treated.

Psychodrama: Psychotherapy wherein clients act out events from their pasts.

Psychoneuroimmunology: The study of mind-body integration, in particular the connections between the psyche, immune system, and central nervous system.

Psychosynthesis: Psychotherapy aiming to integrate separate elements of the psyche.

Pulse diagnosis in TCM: Skilled practitioners feel the radial pulses at both wrists and diagnose the yin/yang balance in twelve meridians. They feel three deep pulses and three superficial pulses on each side.

DR. PETER L. JOHNSTON

Qi Gong: A Chinese system of physical exercises and breathing control related to Tai chi—one that can be directed toward health issues.

Radionics: CAM based on the study of radiation emitted by living matter.

Radiology: The science and practice of using X-rays in medical diagnosis.

Radiotherapy: The use of radiation and nuclear isotopes in medical treatment, mainly in cancer.

Radix body-based psychotherapy: Psychotherapy using postures, exercises, and emotional release techniques. While initiated by Chuck Kelly, it is based on the work of Wilhelm Reich.

Rayid iridology: Denny Johnson found the iris could be used as a map for understanding personality traits and relationship patterns.

Rebirthing: Being able to re-enact the birth process was something Leonard Orr discovered for himself while he was lying in a bath. Later, he found it easier to induce an altered state of consciousness in his clients by using circular breathing and music.

Reflexology: A system of massage used to treat tension and illness. It is based on the theory that there are reflex points on the feet linking with every other part of the body.

Reiki: A form of spiritual healing that uses symbols. Usui, a Japanese spiritualist, found he could activate a person's natural healing potential by touching them. Translated from the Japanese, *reiki* means "universal life energy."

Relationship therapy: What used to be called marriage guidance until marriage ceased to be the sole form of long-term relationships.

Rolfing: A form of deep tissue massage aimed at releasing muscular tension at skeletal level. Named after its initiator, Ida Rolfe, a physiotherapist.

Runes: Alphabet dating possibly from first century. The letters were used to relate to aspects of spiritual and secular life, becoming a magical language used on talismans, inscriptions, and divination.

Sandplay: Psychotherapy using sandboxes, tangible symbols, and gestalt therapy to explore life issues.

Sex therapy: Originating with the work of Masters and Johnson in the 1970s, counselling on sexual dysfunction has become a spe-

THE EAGLE'S WAY

cialty of its own. More recently, the boundaries between sex therapy and relationship counselling have blurred.

Sechem: A form of spiritual healing of Egyptian origin.

Shamanism: A system of healing originating in the tribal cultures of Asia and North America. The shaman or "medicine man" would enter an altered state of consciousness and commune with the spirit world. From there, he would bring back a healing recipe for his client.

Spiritual healing: The term used prior to *reiki* and therapeutic touch. While the familiar form is the "laying on of hands," spiritual healing can also occur without physical touch. Referred to as "absent healing" or "distant healing," people have experienced healing by being sent love and healing intent from another.

Sufi mysticism: A mystic sect of Islam. Famous for their "whirling dervishes," a dance that produces an altered state of consciousness.

Surgery: The branch of medicine involving incisions into the body or repair of wounds.

Tai chi ch'uan: A Chinese system of callisthenics involving sequences of slow, controlled movements. It is like a moving meditation with focus on breath and the movement of the life force (chi).

Tantra: Hindu/Buddhist mystical tradition involving meditation, yoga, and ritual. More popular in the West for its relevance to sexual practice and relationship therapy.

Taoism: Eastern philosophy of Lao Tzu advocating humility and reverence for the natural order of life. In psychotherapy, the phrase "going with the flow" owes much to the wisdom of Taoism.

Tarot cards: A deck of cards popularised by the gypsies who used it for fortune-telling. Possibly dating back to ancient Egypt, the cards may also be helpful in gaining insights into one's character traits.

Therapeutic touch: A form of spiritual healing introduced by Dolores Kreiger. It has become popular with the nursing profession as they can add love and healing intent to the touch they routinely apply to patients.

Tibetan medicine: A holistic model of health care derived from the Tibetan Buddhist culture.

DR. PETER L. JOHNSTON

Thought field therapy (TFT): A meridian-based psychotherapy useful in the treatment of stress, phobias, negative emotions, and addictions.

Tongue diagnosis in TCM: Traditional Chinese medical practitioners can derive a remarkable amount of information about the relative balance of yin and yang just by examining a patient's tongue.

Toning: Wordless singing which not only exercises the vocal chords, but also helps to bring a sense of harmony to the body.

Traditional Chinese medicine (TCM): CAM that can trace its origins back to the *Yellow Emperor's Classic of Internal Medicine*. First published in 1772, it actually refers to the wisdom of the Emperor Huang Ti, who was said to have reigned from 2696 to 2598 BC.

Transactional analysis: Psychotherapeutic system based on Eric Berne's idea that behaviour reflects an interchange between parental, adult, and childlike aspects of personality.

Transpersonal psychology: The study and practice of psychology transcending the boundaries of the physical body.

Twelve-step programs: Alcoholics Anonymous pioneered this system where alcoholics help each other. The same approach is used for gambling and for the partners of alcoholics who tend toward co-dependency.

Ultrasound imaging: Medical system of diagnosis using ultrasound waves. Colour Doppler is a further enhancement of this technique. **Vision quest:** A Native-American custom where people spend time alone in nature getting to know themselves, their purpose, and their
relationship to the Great White Spirit.

Visualisations: Mental images. The New Age has brought about a deeper understanding of the power of visualising one's goals and seeing in detail the successful outcome desired.

Voice dialogue: Psychotherapy devised by Hal and Sidra Stone for communicating with sub-personalities or archetypes.

Weight loss programs: Those that focus on food alone have poor long-term results as most regain lost weight within two years.

Those that include a focus on self-esteem, emotional and psychological factors have more success.

Wholistic hybrid of EMDR and EFT (WHEE): Dr. Dan Benor devised this hybrid, and he has had remarkable success with using it for relieving patient stress and phobias. It is a form of psychotherapy that also focuses on patients loving themselves "wholly, completely, and unconditionally."

Writing with non-dominant hand: Writing with one's left hand if right-handed and vice versa can have the effect of accessing the opposite brain hemisphere.

Yoga: Hindu spiritual and ascetic discipline, a part of which includes breath control, meditation, and the adoption of specific bodily postures called *asanas*. Since the 1960s, yoga has been practised widely in the Western world for health and relaxation.

Zen: Japanese school of Mahayana Buddhism emphasising the value of meditation and intuition. Techniques from Zen are used in psychotherapy to help people "get out of their heads and into their hearts." Zen *koans* can be like paradoxes. They make no sense intellectually.

GLOSSARY OF MEDICAL TERMS

Abscess: A collection of pus in the body.

Acute abdomen: Abdominal pain of sudden onset.

Addison's disease: Disease caused by a deficiency of hormones from adrenal cortex.

AIDS: Acquired immune deficiency syndrome. A disease caused by the HIV virus.

Alzheimer's disease: A common cause of dementia.

Ambulance chaser: A lawyer specialising in personal injury claims.

Amniotic fluid: The fluid or liquor surrounding a baby in the womb.

Anaphylaxis: Extreme allergic reaction to an antigen, producing shock and not infrequently death.

Aneurysm: Localized swelling of an artery. In the brain, a large one can cause pressure and death if it ruptures.

Angina pectoris: Chest pains because of spasms in the coronary arteries.

Angiography: Outlining the blood vessels (or lymphatic vessels) by using X-rays after injecting a radiopaque substance.

Anorectics: Medications used to reduce appetite and lose weight

Anoxia: Oxygen deficiency

Anthelmintics: Drugs used against worm infestations.

Anti-anxiety agents: Drugs used to reduce anxiety.

Anti-arrhythmics: Drugs to combat abnormal heart rhythms.

Antibiotics: Drugs that destroy or inhibit the growth of microorganisms.

THE EAGLE'S WAY

Anticoagulants: Drugs to prevent clotting within the body.

Anticonvulsants: Drugs to prevent and treat epilepsy.

Antidepressants: Medications used to combat depression.

Antidiabetic agents: Drugs to treat diabetes.

Antidiarrhoeals: Drugs to stop or diminish diarrhoea.

Anti-emetics: Drugs used to treat nausea and vomiting.

Antifungals: Drugs used to fight fungal infections.

Antihistamines: Drugs that inhibit the effects of histamine, a body chemical involved in allergic disorders.

Antimetabolites: Drugs used in cancer to interfere with cell metabolism.

Antimigraine drugs: Medications to prevent or ease migraine.

Antineoplastic agents: Drugs used against cancer.

Anti-oxidants: Substances that prevent or inhibit oxidation.

Antiparasitics: Drugs used to combat infestation with parasites.

Anti-Parkinsonian agents: Drugs used in the treatment of Parkinson's disease.

Antipsychotic agents: Drugs used for the treatment of psychoses, especially schizophrenia.

Antispasmodics: Drugs used to relieve smooth muscle spasm in hollow organs.

Appendicitis: Inflammation of the appendix.

Arthritis: Inflammation of joints.

Atropine: A drug derived from deadly nightshade plants and used to dry up secretions.

Bacteria: Single-celled microorganisms, some of which are helpful to metabolic functions (commensals), others harmful (pathogenic).

Beriberi: Disease caused by lack of vitamin B1 (thiamine).

Blastema: A mass of undifferentiated cells capable of growth and regeneration into organs.

Blepharospasm: Involuntary tight closure of the eyelids.

Breech birth: When the baby arrives buttocks-first rather than the usual headfirst.

Cachexia: Weakness and wasting of the body because of severe chronic illness.

Capillaries: Microscopic blood vessels forming a network and linking blood flow between the smaller arteries and veins.

345

Carcinogens/carcinogenic: Cancer-producing agents.

Cardiologist: A specialist in heart disease.

Cardiopulmonary resuscitation (CPR): Combination of chest compression and mouth-to mouth resuscitation in patients who have gone into cardiac arrest.

Cardiovascular events: Those affecting heart and blood vessels. Usually refers to heart attacks or strokes.

Cataract: Opacity in the optic lens.

Catharsis: The process of releasing pent-up emotions.

Cerebral palsy: A condition caused by brain damage prior to or during birth.

Chronic fatigue syndrome: A disease of unknown cause characterised by prolonged fatigue and exhaustion together with muscle aches and pains.

Cirrhosis: Chronic disease of the liver following hepatitis or chronic alcoholism.

Coccyx: Small triangular bone at base of spinal column.

Convulsions: Violent, uncontrolled body movements caused by toxins or epilepsy.

Coronaries: The arteries to the heart.

Coronary Bypass: Surgery to bypass blocked arteries and allow unimpeded circulation to the heart.

Corpus callosum: A broad band of nerve fibres linking the left and right hemispheres of the brain.

Corticosteroids: Hormones secreted from the cortex of the adrenal gland.

Crohn's disease (regional ileitis): Inflammatory disease of the small bowel—sometimes found in large bowel as well.

Croup: Viral inflammation of the larynx and trachea in children.

Cyanotic: Bluish colour of lips and skin due to lack of adequate oxygen perfusion.

Cystitis—Inflammation of the urinary bladder.

Deep vein thrombosis (DVT): Clotting in deep veins, usually in lower limbs or pelvis; associated with stasis as in long operations or aircraft flights.

THE EAGLE'S WAY

Defibrillation: The application of an electric shock to treat ventricular fibrillation, a lethal arrhythmia of the heart. A successful treatment will restore normal rhythm.

Delirium: Acutely disturbed state of mind characterised by restlessness, confusion, and illusions, occurring in fever, intoxication, and other toxic states.

Delusion: A belief that is inconsistent with generally accepted reality.

Dementia: Chronic brain disorder affecting memory, behaviour, and reasoning.

Dermatologist: Skin specialist.

Diabetes mellitus: Disease caused by deficiency of insulin, a pancreatic hormone.

Dialysis: A process of blood cleansing replacing the function of kidneys. Sometimes referred to as "artificial kidney."

Disc degeneration: Degeneration of the cartilaginous cushions between the vertebral bones in the spine.

Diverticulae: Abnormal pouches formed at weak points in the wall of the large bowel. When inflamed, becomes diverticulitis.

DNA: Deoxyribonucleic acid, the double-stranded chemical that carries the genes.

Down's syndrome: A congenital disorder causing intellectual impairment and characteristic physical features.

Duodenal ulcer: Erosion in the internal lining of the duodenum, which is the first part of the small bowel. Sometimes referred to as peptic ulcer.

Emphysema: Chronic lung disease, frequently the result of smoking.

Encephalitis: Viral infection of the brain.

Endocrinologist: Specialist in diseases of the endocrine glands.

Femur: Thigh bone including part of the hip.

Fibre optics: The use of thin flexible transparent fibres to transmit light.

Fibrotic lung disease: Chronic disease characterised by thickening of lung tissue.

Gallstones: Hard masses formed in the gall bladder from bile, calcium, or cholesterol.

Gamma waves: brainwave frequencies which signify the highest state of focus possible. They are associated with optimal cognitive functioning.

Gastroenteritis: Inflammation of the digestive tract.

Gastroenterologist: Specialist in diseases of the digestive tract.

Gastrointestinal: The digestive tract from oesophagus (gullet) to anus.

Glomerulonephritis: Inflammation of the kidney, usually because of an immune response.

Haematologist: Specialist in diseases of the blood.

Haemophilia: A disorder in which the clotting capacity of the body is impaired.

Haemostasis: Tying off blood vessels to stop bleeding.

Hallucination: An experience of something not visible to others in the same physical space.

Hemi-corporectomy: Removal of half of the body.

Hepatitis: Inflammation of the liver, usually viral in origin.

Heterograft: A graft taken from another person, living or deceased.

HIV positive: A positive pathology test showing the presence of the HIV virus.

Homograft: A graft taken from another area of the patient's anatomy. **Huntington's disease:** Hereditary disease of the brain and nervous system characterised by involuntary movements and progressive dementia.

Hypertension: High blood pressure.

Hypnosis: An altered state of consciousness characterised by high responsiveness.

Hypothyroidism: Under activity of the thyroid gland.

Iatrogenic: Of or pertaining to illness caused by medical treatment.

Ideopathic: A disease for which the cause is unknown.

Immunisation: Rendering the body immune to specific infections by inoculation.

In vitro: Taking place outside the body—in a test-tube or culture dish.

Influenza: Highly infectious viral infection of respiratory passages. To be differentiated from the milder common cold, affecting the same passages.

THE EAGLE'S WAY

Ipecac: A drug derived from the South American shrub *ipecacuanha* and used to induce vomiting, most often in cases of attempted suicide from drug over dosage.

Iris: The coloured part of the eye around the pupil.

Irritable bowel syndrome: A condition characterised by abdominal pain and bowel disturbances, usually related to stress.

IV fluids: Electrolytes and liquids administered through veins.

JVP: Jugular venous pressure. This is raised in patients with heart failure.

Ketosis: Excess ketones in body caused by fat metabolism, especially in diabetes.

Killer cells: Cells of the immune system whose role is to kill cancer cells.

Kadaitcha: In Central Aboriginal tribes, the man with the mission of avenging the death of a tribesman (*Collins Australian Dictionary*).

Leboyer delivery: Gentle natural birth using soft music and water immersion.

Lens (Optic): The transparent elastic structure behind the iris by which light is focused on the retina.

Ligand: A small triggering molecule that binds onto a site on a target protein.

LSD: Lysergic acid diethylamide, a recreational drug with hallucinogenic capacity.

Lumbar: The lower back area

Lymphoma: Cancer in lymph nodes, Hodgkin's being the most common.

Macular degeneration: Degeneration of the macula, the central area in the retina, which is the area of greatest visual acuity.

Malarial parasite: A protozoan of genus *plasmodium,* causing malaria.

Melanoma: A malignant tumour deriving from pigment cells in the skin.

Meningitis: Inflammation of the membranes surrounding the spinal cord and brain.

Meprobamate: A drug used for anxiety. First manufactured in 1955. Used less now.

Metabolism: Chemical processes occurring within the body in order to maintain life.

Metastatic cancer: Secondary tumours arising at a distance from the original primary site of cancer.

Migraine: Severe headache affecting one side of the head only. Often accompanied by nausea, vomiting and aversion to light. Sometimes other neurological symptoms.

Mitochondria: components of the cell that convert glucose into energy.

Modality: A method or procedure.

Mogadon: A sleeping tablet of the benzodiazepine group.

Morbidity: Disease.

Morphine: A narcotic derived from opium and used to relieve severe pain.

Morphogenetic fields: Non-physical blueprints that give rise to form. A concept formed in 1973 by Rupert Shedrake, a biologist.

Motor neurone disease: A disease characterised by progressive wasting and paralysis of muscles.

Multiple sclerosis: Disease of unknown origin characterised by loss of myelin in the nervous system. It frequently affects young adults.

Nephrologist: Specialist in diseases of the kidney. **Neural:** Of or pertaining to a nerve or the nervous system. **Neurologist:** Specialist in diseases of the nervous system.

Neuropeptide: One of a group of polypeptide compounds, which act as neurotransmitters.

Neurosurgeon: Brain and spinal cord surgeon.

Obstetrics: Pertaining to childbirth.

Ophthalmologist: Eye specialist.

Opiate receptor: Tissue in the cell wall that responds to derivatives of opium.

Optic cortex: The area of the brain associated with visual storage and processing.

Orthopaedic surgeon: Surgeon specialising in bone and joint surgery.

Osteomyelitis: Inflammation of bone.

Osteoporosis: Thinning of density of bone resulting in fragility and fractures.

Otosclerosis: Hereditary disease of the middle ear leading to progressive deafness.

Ovarian cyst: Fluid-filled sac in the ovary. It can rupture, causing abdominal pain.

Palliative: Alleviating a problem without dealing with the cause.

Pancreatic enzymes: Enzymes that are produced in the pancreas and secreted directly into the duodenum to aid digestion.

Pancreatitis: Inflammation of the pancreas.

Panhypopituitarism: Under activity of the pituitary gland.

Paranormal: Phenomena or events that are considered beyond the scope of normal scientific understanding.

Parathyroids: Glands in the neck producing hormones that regulate calcium levels in the body.

Parkinson's disease: A progressive disease of the brain characterised by tremor, muscular rigidity, and slow, imprecise movement.

Pathogen: A microorganism capable of causing disease.

Pathology: The study of disease.

Pathology tests: Those looking for disease.

Penicillin: An antibiotic originating from the mould *penicillium notatum.*

Peptic ulcer: An erosion of the lining of the stomach or duodenum because of excessive concentration or action of acidic digestive enzymes.

Perforated peptic ulcer: Erosion of ulcer deep enough to fully penetrate wall of stomach or duodenum.

Pethidine: Narcotic pain reliever in the opiate group.

Phenylketonuria: An inherited inability to metabolise the amino acid, phenylalanine, the lack of which can bring about brain and nerve damage.

Phobia: An irrational or excessive fear of something.

Physiology: The study of bodily function in health.

Pituitary: A gland at the base of the brain that produces hormones controlling all the other endocrine glands.

Pneumonia: Infection in the lungs.

Prolapsed cord: Umbilical cord emerging from the womb prior to birth of baby.

Protozoa: Single-celled organisms like amoebae.

Pulmonary embolus: Life-threatening blood clots in lungs usually arising secondary to deep vein thrombosis.

Pulmonary hypertension: High blood pressure in the arteries flowing to the lungs.

Rabies: Viral infection affecting dogs and other mammals, including humans, leading to convulsions and insanity.

Respiratory physician: Specialist in diseases of the lungs and respiratory tract.

Retina: The light-sensitive membrane on the back surface of the eye.

Rhesus factor: Antigen on blood cells, noted as positive or negative in everyone's blood group.

Rheumatoid arthritis: Chronic progressive inflammatory disease involving joints.

Rubella: A viral infection otherwise known as German measles.

Ruptured ectopic: A pregnancy in the fallopian tube, which has burst.

Sac: A bag formed of membrane. Used here in reference to the sac of fluid surrounding a baby while in the womb.

Schistosomiasis (bilharzia): A chronic disease endemic in parts of Africa and South America caused by infestation with blood flukes (schistosomes).

Scurvy: Disease caused by vitamin C deficiency.

Seldinger technique: A procedure to obtain safe access to blood vessels and hollow organs.

Septicaemia: Infection in the bloodstream.

Serepax: A tranquilliser of the benzodiazepine group.

Sickle cell anaemia: An inherited trait producing a lack of oxygen in the red blood cells, causing them to change into a sickle-like shape.

SSRIs: A group of antidepressant medications.

Strangulated hernia: Hernia is a condition in which a part of the bowel protrudes through a weakness in the abdominal wall. Strangulation occurs when its circulation is cut off, usually by a twisting of the bowel within the hernia.

Streptomycin: Antibiotic mainly used against tuberculosis.

Sulphonamides: A group of drugs capable of inhibiting the reproduction of bacteria.

Syndrome: A collection of symptoms and signs that consistently occur together.

Syphilis: A sexually transmitted bacterial disease capable of progressing to cause chronic lesions in the heart, brain, and almost any organ in the body.

Systemic lupus erythematosis (SLE): An auto-immune disease affecting multiple organs.

T-cells: Cells of the immune system produced originally in the thymus gland.

Tennis elbow: Medically known as "epicondylitis," it is a common, painful inflammation of the lateral part of the elbow at the origin of the extensor tendons.

Tenosynovitis: Inflammation of a tendon most commonly in the wrist.

Toxicity: A state of being poisoned.

Transpersonal: Pertaining to states of consciousness beyond the limits of personal identity.

Tricuspid incompetence: A malfunction of the valve in the right side of the heart.

Tricyclics: A group of drugs used in the treatment of depression.

Tuberculosis (TB): A bacterial disease characterised by the growth of nodules in the tissues, especially in the lungs.

Ulcerative colitis: Inflammatory disease affecting large bowel.

Ureteric calculi: Hard masses that have formed in the kidneys and moved down into the ureter where they cannot pass easily and thereby cause severe pain.

Urologist: Surgeon specialising in the urinary tract.

Vaccination: Originating from the treatment of smallpox with vaccinia virus, it is now being used as a synonym for immunisation.

Valium: A tranquilliser of the benzodiazepine group.

Ventolin: Medication used to relieve the bronchospasm of asthma

Villi: Finger-like projections lining small intestine that help absorption.

Virus: A sub-microscopic microorganism causing dise

Printed in the USA
CPSIA information can be obtained
at www.ICGtesting.com
LVHW091941041023
760094LV00001B/99